Pediatric Rehabilitation

Editor

ANDREW J. SKALSKY

PHYSICAL MEDICINE AND REHABILITATION CLINICS OF NORTH AMERICA

www.pmr.theclinics.com

Consulting Editor
GREGORY T. CARTER

February 2015 • Volume 26 • Number 1

ELSEVIER

1600 John F. Kennedy Boulevard • Suite 1800 • Philadelphia, Pennsylvania, 19103-2899

http://www.theclinics.com

PHYSICAL MEDICINE AND REHABILITATION CLINICS OF NORTH AMERICA Volume 26, Number 1
February 2015 ISSN 1047-9651, ISBN 978-0-323-35449-3

Editor: Jennifer Flynn-Briggs
Developmental Editor: Don Mumford

Reprints. For copies of 100 or more of articles in this publication, please contact the Commercial Reprints Department, Elsevier Inc., 360 Park Avenue South, New York, NY 10010-1710. Tel.: 212-633-3874; Fax: 212-633-3820; E-mail: reprints@elsevier.com.

Physical Medicine and Rehabilitation Clinics of North America (ISSN 1047-9651) is published quarterly by Elsevier Inc., 360 Park Avenue South, New York, NY 10010-1710. Months of issue are February, May, August, and November. Business and Editorial Offices: 1600 John F. Kennedy Blvd., Suite 1800, Philadelphia, PA 19103-2899. Customer Service Office: 3251 Riverport Lane, Maryland Heights, MO 63043. Periodicals postage paid at New York, NY and additional mailing offices. Subscription price per year is $275.00 (US individuals), $486.00 (US institutions), $145.00 (US students), $335.00 (Canadian individuals), $640.00 (Canadian institutions), $210.00 (Canadian students), $415.00 (foreign individuals), $640.00 (foreign institutions), and $210.00 (foreign students). Foreign air speed delivery is included in all *Clinics* subscription prices. All prices are subject to change without notice. **POSTMASTER:** Send address changes to *Physical Medicine and Rehabilitation Clinics of North America*, Customer Service Office: Elsevier Health Sciences Division, Subscription Customer Service, 3251 Riverport Lane, Maryland Heights, MO 63043. **Customer Service: 1-800-654-2452 (US). From outside of the United States, call 314-447-8871. Fax: 314-447-8029. E-mail: JournalsCustomer Service-usa@elsevier.com (for print support); JournalsOnlineSupport-usa@elsevier.com (for online support).**

Physical Medicine and Rehabilitation Clinics of North America is indexed in *Excerpta Medica, MEDLINE/PubMed (Index Medicus), Cinahl,* and *Cumulative Index to Nursing and Allied Health Literature.*

Contributors

CONSULTING EDITOR

GREGORY T. CARTER, MD, MS
Consulting Medical Editor, Medical Director, St Luke's Rehabilitation Institute, Spokane, Washington; University of Washington, School of Medicine, Seattle, Washington

EDITOR

ANDREW J. SKALSKY, MD
Assistant Professor, Division of Pediatric Rehabilitation Medicine, Department of Pediatrics; Chief of Rehabilitation Medicine, Rady Children's Hospital San Diego, University of California San Diego, San Diego, California

AUTHORS

HENRY G. CHAMBERS, MD
Professor of Clinical Orthopedic Surgery, Director of Cerebral Palsy Program, Rady Children's Hospital, San Diego, University of California San Diego, San Diego, California

JILL A. CHAMBERS, CHTP
Rady Children's Hospital, San Diego, San Diego, California

PRITHA B. DALAL, MD
Associate Physician, Division of Pediatric Rehabilitation Medicine, Department of Pediatrics, Rady Children's Hospital San Diego, University of California San Diego, San Diego, California

LOREN DAVIDSON, MD
Associate Professor, Department of Physical Medicine and Rehabilitation, Shriners Hospitals for Children — Northern California; University of California Davis Health System, Sacramento, California

CHRYSTAL M. FOURNIER, MSN, RN, FNP-BC
Division of Pediatric Rehabilitation Medicine, Rady Children's Hospital San Diego, San Diego, California

JOAN T. LE, MD
Associate Physician, Division of Pediatric Rehabilitation Medicine, Department of Pediatrics, Rady Children's Hospital San Diego, University of California San Diego, San Diego, California

DANIEL J. LESSER, MD
Assistant Professor, Division of Pediatric Respiratory Medicine, Department of Pediatrics, Rady Children's Hospital San Diego, University of California San Diego, San Diego, California

RICHARD L. LIEBER, PhD
Departments of Orthopaedic Surgery, University of California San Diego, La Jolla, California; Department of Veteran's Affairs, San Diego, California

MARGIE A. MATHEWSON, PhD
Department of Bioengineering, University of California San Diego, La Jolla, California

CRAIG M. McDONALD, MD
Professor, Department of Physical Medicine and Rehabilitation, University of California Davis School of Medicine, Davis, California

SHUBHRA MUKHERJEE, MD, FRCPC
Pediatric and Adolescent Rehabilitation Medicine, Rehabilitation Institute of Chicago, Ann and Robert H. Lurie Children's Hospital of Chicago Spina Bifida Clinic, Northwestern University Feinberg School of Medicine, Chicago, Illinois

WENDY PIERCE, MD
Assistant Professor, Department of Physical Medicine and Rehabilitation, University of Colorado, Colorado Springs, Colorado

AARON POWELL, MD
Department of Physical Medicine and Rehabilitation, University of California Davis Medical Center, University of California Davis Health System, Sacramento, California

GINA REMPEL, MD, FRCPC, FAAP
Chief Medical Officer, Rehabilitation Centre for Children, Inc, Winnipeg, Manitoba, Canada; Associate Professor of Pediatrics and Child Health, University of Manitoba; Medical Director of the Feeding Eating and Swallowing Teams (FEAST), Children's Hospital and Rehabilitation Centre for Children, and the Pediatric Manitoba Home Nutrition Program, Winnipeg, Canada

BRIAN SCANNELL, MD
Assistant Professor, Department of Orthopaedics, Levine Children's Hospital, Carolinas Medical Center, Charlotte, North Carolina

PHOEBE R. SCOTT-WYARD, DO
Medical Director, Child Amputee Prosthetics Project, Shriners Hospital - Los Angeles; Staff Physician, Pediatric Rehabilitation Division, Children's Hospital Los Angeles, Los Angeles, California

ANDREW J. SKALSKY, MD
Assistant Professor, Division of Pediatric Rehabilitation Medicine, Department of Pediatrics; Chief of Rehabilitation Medicine, Rady Children's Hospital San Diego, University of California San Diego, San Diego, California

ANNE STRATTON, MD
Assistant Professor, Department of Physical Medicine and Rehabilitation, University of Colorado, Denver, Colorado

SATHYA VADIVELU, MD
Division of Pediatric Rehabilitation Medicine, Department of Pediatrics, Rady Children's Hospital San Diego, University of California San Diego, San Diego, California

BURT YASZAY, MD
Clinical Assistant Professor, Department of Pediatric Orthopaedics, Rady Children's Hospital San Diego, San Diego, California

Contents

> Parents of children with disabilities encounter stresses unlike those of families with typically developing children. Medical professionals must appreciate that they are not only treating the child but also the family. A state-of-the-art understanding of their patient's disability is implied, but they must also understand the dynamics of raising a child with a disability, appreciate the different models of health care delivery, and provide guidance in transition to adulthood in healthcare as well as life (education, living arrangements, conservancy, etc). An awareness of the physical and mental health impacts on the parents of a child with a chronic disability should also be appreciated.

> Children with pediatric neuromuscular disorders experience common complications, primarily due to immobility and weakness. Musculoskeletal complications include hip dysplasia with associated hip subluxation or dislocation, neuromuscular scoliosis, and osteoporosis and resulting fractures. Constipation, gastroesophageal reflux, and obesity and malnutrition are commonly experienced gastrointestinal complications. Disordered sleep also is frequently observed, which affects both patients and caregivers.

> More individuals with spina bifida are living into adulthood, and unique challenges arise as they age. These patients have multiple organ system involvement in addition to physical impairments, disabilities, cognitive involvement, and psychosocial challenges. There is a growing need for transitional care for adults with spina bifida. This article explores the 5 key elements for a transition program to adult care: preparation, flexible timing, care coordination, transitional clinic visits, and health care providers who are interested in taking care of adults with disabilities.

Intrathecal baclofen (ITB), administered by an implanted pump, has emerged as an efficacious therapy for the treatment of hypertonicity in pediatrics. Although ITB has been used for more than 20 years clinically, much is still unknown about the most optimal dosing regimens and intrathecal catheter tip placement. Clinician experience, animal research, and advanced imaging is guiding the use of ITB. The rationale for high cervical catheter tip placement and pulsating flex dosing is described.

Congenital limb differences are uncommon birth defects that may go undetected even with prenatal screening ultrasound scans and often go undetected until birth. For children with congenital limb differences, a diagnostic evaluation should be done to rule out syndromes involving other organ systems or known associations. The most common etiology of acquired amputation is trauma. Postamputation complications include pain and terminal bony overgrowth. A multidisciplinary approach to management with the child and family can lead to a successful, functional, and fulfilling life.

 Video of tendon transfer surgery accompanies this article

In this article, an overview is provided of pediatric spinal cord injury, organized by effects of this injury on various organ systems. Specific management differences between children and adults with spinal cord injury are highlighted. A detailed management approach is offered for particularly complex topics, such as spasticity and upper extremity reconstruction.

Assessing phrenic nerve function in the setting of diaphragmatic paralysis in diaphragm pacing candidates can be challenging. Traditional imaging modalities and electrodiagnostic evaluations are technically difficult. Either modality alone is not a direct measure of the function of the phrenic nerve and diaphragm unit. In this article, the authors present their method for evaluating phrenic nerve function and the resulting diaphragm function. Stimulating the phrenic nerve with transcutaneous stimulation and directly observing the resulting movement of the hemidiaphragm with M-mode ultrasonography provides quantitative data for predicting the success of advancing technologies such as phrenic nerve pacing and diaphragm pacing.

PHYSICAL MEDICINE AND REHABILITATION CLINICS OF NORTH AMERICA

VISIT THE CLINICS ONLINE!
Access your subscription at:
www.theclinics.com

DOWNLOAD
Free App!

Review Articles
THE CLINICS

NOW AVAILABLE FOR YOUR iPhone and iPad

Foreword

Pediatric Rehabilitation

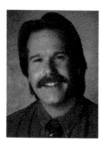

Gregory T. Carter, MD, MS
Consulting Editor

In the scope of medicine overall, and even within our own specialty of Physical Medicine and Rehabilitation, children with disabilities represent a unique population. Pediatric rehabilitation may be the most challenging subspecialty within our field as it focuses on maximizing the function and enhancing the lives of children with a wide range of conditions such as cerebral palsy, spina bifida, stroke, brain injury, genetic abnormalities, and other developmental disabilities. As with adult rehabilitation, it is a multidisciplinary venture and it takes a certain type of personality to be able to do this. Not only are you dealing with a disabled child, but also you are dealing with parents and other family members. Despite a growing need, there is a huge shortage of fully trained pediatric physiatrists. Thus, many of us who are primarily trained in adult physiatry end up doing some of this. Thus, this issue of *Physical Medicine and Rehabilitation Clinics of North America* becomes even more important.

I have known our guest editor, Dr Andrew Skalsky, since he was in training at the University of California, Davis. From the start, it was clear that Andrew was going to be a leader in the field. He is very driven, highly intelligent, and visionary. I had no hesitation in asking Andrew to do this project. In fact, he came immediately to mind. I knew Andrew would come through for us and indeed he has.

Starting us off is an excellent article entitled, "The Importance of Good Nutrition in Children with Cerebral Palsy," by Dr Gina Rempel, Chief Medical Officer of the Rehabilitation Centre for Children Pediatrics and Child Health, Winnipeg, University of Manitoba. She is the Director of Feeding Services at Children's Hospital and Rehabilitation Centre for Children and the Pediatric Medical Director of the Manitoba Home Nutrition Program. This article defines guidelines to maximize nutrition in this fragile population.

My colleagues from the University of California, Davis, Drs Aaron Powell and Loren Davidson, provide a very thorough update on Pediatric Spinal Cord Injury. This article is organized by organ system effects, which makes it very easy to read and provides guidelines that any practicing clinician can use.

Phys Med Rehabil Clin N Am 26 (2015) ix–xi
http://dx.doi.org/10.1016/j.pmr.2014.10.004
1047-9651/15/$ – see front matter © 2015 Elsevier Inc. All rights reserved.

The complex topic of "Scoliosis, Spinal Fusion, and Intrathecal Baclofen Pump Implantation" is covered in detail by pediatric orthopedic specialists from Rady Children's Hospital in San Diego, Drs Brian Scannell and Burt Yaszay. Readers will find this area nicely broken down into usable clinical guidelines and recommendations.

A very compelling and thoughtful article entitled, "Effects of Caregiving on the Families of Children and Adults with Disabilities," is provided by Henry G. Chambers, MD and Jill A. Chambers, CHTP. I found this article to provide very useful guidelines for the overall management of this very challenging population. There is good discussion of the multifaceted psychosocial challenges that often arise and may be very hard to deal with in a clinical scenario.

My good friend and colleague, Dr Rick Lieber, along with Margie A. Mathewson, MS, provide us with an excellent article entitled, "Pathophysiology of Muscle Contractures in Cerebral Palsy." Even ambulatory children with cerebral palsy may present with contractures, often compounded by abnormal gait patterns due to muscular spasticity. This article really delves into the underlying processes that can lead to this and proves a scientific basis for further study on how to prevent disabling contractures in this population. Rick has recently been appointed Senior Vice President of Research and Chief Scientist at the Rehabilitation Institute of Chicago, a hugely important position at our nation's largest and preeminent rehabilitation hospital. I wish him well in this new role and I am certain he will be successful.

Pediatric rehabilitation specialists, Drs Joan T. Le and Phoebe R. Scott-Wyard, provide an outstanding update on "Pediatric Limb Differences and Amputation." The pediatric amputee population can be very challenging and preservation of maximal limb length during amputation may not always be possible. This article provides a thorough discussion of how to maximize the efficiency and symmetry of function, including gait. The authors provide thoughtful discussion of functional outcomes given various levels of amputation and limb loss.

Dr Le, along with colleague Dr Shubhra Mukherjee, authored "Transition to Adult Care for Patients with Spina Bifida." I think this area is very challenging, particularly when it comes to identifying the critical areas of need that must be closely followed as adolescents become adult patients with spina bifida. Many areas, such as urologic care, could pose life-threatening problems if not adequately addressed. I applaud the authors for a very comprehensive discussion of how this should occur. Delays in transition to adult care are known to be associated with higher rates of comorbidity.

"Common Complications of Pediatric Neuromuscular Disorders" is authored by Drs Skalsky and Pritha B. Dalal. For all of these disorders, there may be a plethora of problems, and it is critical to identify them early on and take a proactive management course. This article provides a tactical approach for doing this.

Dr Skalsky, along with pediatric pulmonologist, Dr Daniel J. Lesser, from Rady Children's Hospital, and my close friend and colleague, Dr Craig M. McDonald, from UC Davis do an excellent job of covering the complex topic of phrenic nerve pacing. They provide us an article entitled, "Evaluation of Phrenic Nerve and Diaphragm Function with Peripheral Nerve Stimulation and M-Mode Ultrasonography in Potential Pediatric Phrenic Nerve or Diaphragm Pacing Candidates."

Dr Skalsky, MD and Chrystal M. Fournier, MSN, RN, FNP-BC close out this issue with an article entitled, "Intrathecal Baclofen Bolus Dosing and Catheter Tip Placement in Pediatric Tone Management," which goes into detail on management strategies to ensure the best outcome for those children affected by motor control disorders that can accompany the long-term effects of disorders like cerebral palsy, traumatic brain injury, and a myriad of neurologic disorders. Proper tone management with a baclofen pump can have a positive effect on issues such as standing ability, gait, and even other muscular issues such as bladder control.

As always, I want to express my sincerest gratitude to all of these renowned authors for the efforts they have put forth here in providing us with another exceptional issue of the *Physical Medicine and Rehabilitation Clinics of North America* series. I would like to extend a special measure of gratitude to our guest editor, and my good friend, Dr Andrew Skalsky, for leading this project and giving us such a superb and timely update on major issues in pediatric rehabilitation. These authors have given us a directly useful and highly valuable addition to the series.

Gregory T. Carter, MD, MS
St Luke's Rehabilitation Institute
711 South Cowley Street
Spokane, WA 99202, USA

E-mail address:
gtcarter@uw.edu

Preface

Pediatric Rehabilitation

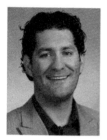

Andrew J. Skalsky, MD
Editor

I am very honored to be the guest editor of this issue of *Physical Medicine and Rehabilitation Clinics of North America* on pediatric rehabilitation. The subspecialty of Pediatric Rehabilitation Medicine is a very small group with just over 200 board-certified specialists in North America. There are over 500,000 children in North America with cerebral palsy and more than 10,000 babies born each year will develop cerebral palsy, not to mention the other diagnoses commonly seen by pediatric physiatrists.

As a result, I feel I have an obligation as a pediatric rehabilitation specialist to not only treat my own patients but also help empower my colleagues to provide more optimal care for children suffering from pediatric-onset physical impairments to maximize their function and quality of life. For this issue of *Physical Medicine and Rehabilitation Clinics of North America*, my goal was to provide a combination of topics that are well known to most pediatric physiatrists yet remain relatively nebulous to pediatricians and other pediatric specialties. In addition, I have tried to highlight some important treatment principles that, despite not being novel, have not been widely adapted despite the growing body of evidence and outcomes to support their use. Although there is a paucity of evidence-based literature relative to the care needs

Phys Med Rehabil Clin N Am 26 (2015) xiii–xiv
http://dx.doi.org/10.1016/j.pmr.2014.10.002
1047-9651/15/$ – see front matter © 2015 Elsevier Inc. All rights reserved.

of our patients, we can positively impact the lives of patients and their families drastically.

I want to thank all of the contributing authors for their hard work and dedication not only to this issue but also to their patients and families and to the field of pediatric rehabilitation.

Andrew J. Skalsky, MD
Chief of Rehabilitation Medicine
Rady Children's Hospital San Diego
3020 Children's Way, MC 5096
San Diego, CA 92123, USA

E-mail address:
askalsky@rchsd.org

Dedication

This issue is dedicated to Dr David Kilmer. Although his time with us was tragically cut short, the knowledge and approach to medicine I gained from his teaching, expertise, and attitude are timeless. I was a trainee in his department, where he passed on much wisdom, which at the time seemed unnecessary and unessential, especially as I prepared for board examinations and certifications. I have since been repeatedly amazed at how valuable and accurate his insight and guidance have proven to be. I recall one specific scenario where he offered his sagely advise, unfortunately, after he had become quite ill. I was in a situation many of us have faced in pediatric rehabilitation medicine where the need was great, but the resources were limited. Although I was complaining, his response was quite clear and profound, "Then there is much need for you there and the children will be very fortunate for your care. You went into medicine to help others, and this sounds like a great opportunity to do just that." Thank-you, Dave, for the bigger lessons you taught me that cannot be acquired from a textbook.

With perpetual gratitude,

Andrew J. Skalsky, MD
Chief of Rehabilitation Medicine
Rady Children's Hospital San Diego
3020 Children's Way, MC 5096
San Diego, CA 92123, USA

E-mail address:
askalsky@rchsd.org

Phys Med Rehabil Clin N Am 26 (2015) xv
http://dx.doi.org/10.1016/j.pmr.2014.10.003
1047-9651/15/$ – see front matter © 2015 Elsevier Inc. All rights reserved.

Effects of Caregiving on the Families of Children and Adults with Disabilities

Henry G. Chambers, MD[a],*, Jill A. Chambers, CHTP[b]

KEYWORDS

- Chronic disability • Quality of life • Caregivers

KEY POINTS

- There are a host of physical and mental stressors in caring for a child with a chronic disability.
- The child and the family progress through different medical aspects of their disorder, but also through different aspects of life.
- There are different models of care provision that can impact the family's overall well-being.
- There are simple methods to interact with families that will increase their satisfaction and happiness.
- There are multiple challenges in transition and care of adults with disabilities.

INTRODUCTION

Medical professionals must remember that they are not only treating the child with a disability, they are also treating the family. The diagnosis of a disability for their child is usually one of the most unexpected and life-altering revelations in a family's life. It is the responsibility of the medical care professional to not only have the state-of-the-art understanding of the child's diagnosis and treatment, but also to appreciate the impact and implications of this diagnosis on the family.[1] There are over 6 million children in the United States with severe disabilities and nearly all of them are cared for at home.[2]

There are a host of physical and mental health problems in caregivers of children and adults with chronic disabilities. The consequences of impaired caregiver health include recurrent hospitalizations for their children[3] and the decision to place their child outside of the home.[4,5]

The authors have nothing to disclose.

[a] Rady Children's Hospital, San Diego, University of California San Diego, 3030 Children's Way, Suite 410, San Diego, CA 92123, USA; [b] Rady Children's Hospital, San Diego, San Diego, CA, USA
* Corresponding author.
E-mail address: hchambers@rchsd.org

- Seventy percent of mothers of children with physical disabilities have low back pain.[6]
- There is a higher incidence of migraine headaches, gastrointestinal ulcers, and greater overall distress.[7]
- Parents report more anxiety, anger, guilt, frustration, sorrow, social isolation, self-deprivation, and depression.

Murphy and colleagues,[8] in an excellent review and utilizing a focus group methodology determined 5 themes that encapsulate the caregivers' experiences:

- Stress of caregiving,
- Negative impact on caregiver health,
- Sharing the burden,
- Worry about the future, and
- Caregiver coping strategies.

GIVING AND GETTING THE DIAGNOSIS

Getting the diagnosis of a chronic disability is obviously a life-changing event. Parents assume that their children will always be "normal" or developing typically. Many parents, of course, have already observed that their child is different from other children their age. They have sought medical care to help make the diagnosis. Diagnoses such as cerebral palsy, muscular dystrophy, and autism, for example, are not usually diagnosed at birth. Patients with obvious birth defects and congenital anomalies are diagnosed at birth, but the parents are anxious for diagnosis and prognosis. There is a different dynamic in diagnosing acquired disabilities, such as spinal cord injury and traumatic brain injury.

Antonak and Livneh[9] describe the stages of a family's response to the diagnosis of a disability. They suggested that there was a 3-cluster approach that involves 8 phases that often unfold sequentially:

- Early reactions of shock, anxiety, and denial;
- Intermediate reactions of depression, internalized anger, and externalized hostility; and
- Later reactions with knowledge and adjustment.

Within each of these processes, there are an additional 4 classes of variables: Those associated with the disability, variables associated with sociodemographic characteristics, and variables associated with physical and social environmental factors. It is therefore difficult as a diagnosing physician to determine what stage of acceptance of the disability that the family is currently in, as well as to understand the personalities of the family and the child. There are families who stay in a stage of denial for years, whereas others rapidly accept the facts before them and move on to the treatment phase. Sociodemographic factors can include the fact that men and women approach the same events differently. There are certainly many cultural differences affecting how a person approaches disabilities. Although complex, it is the role of the physician and the treatment team to ascertain where on this continuum the family lies.[10]

FACTORS OF PARENTING A CHILD WITH A DISABILITY

Peshawaria in an unpublished presentation in 2000 suggests that there are several domains of parenting a child with a disability. These include physical care, health, employment or career, support in the community, financial considerations, social embarrassment, relationships of the child and the family, and the effects of the disability on siblings. Each individual child within each individual disability presents unique physical care challenges. Certainly a child who has a diagnosis of gross motor function classification system (GMFCS) level I cerebral palsy is completely different from a child with GMFCS level V cerebral palsy. A 2-year-old boy with Duchenne muscular dystrophy is also completely different from a 20-year-old boy with the same diagnosis.

RAISING A CHILD WITH A DISABILITY

Raising a typically developing child is difficult enough for most families. However, the parents of a child with a disability, in addition to being faced with the shock of the diagnosis of the disability itself, encounter a host of new challenges. The families are learning new medical terms, such as cerebral palsy, muscular dystrophy, necrotizing enterocolitis, and a myriad of concepts that are probably foreign to them. Agencies such as United Cerebral Palsy, the Muscular Dystrophy Association, the Spina Bifida Association, and other disability service groups can provide significant resources in the early diagnosis phase as well as throughout the child's life. These groups provide education, support, and in some cases hands-on treatment. The family learns a new vocabulary of government agencies and programs with complicated acronyms, rules, and forms.

A newborn or any child with a medical problem can significantly impact the family dynamics. Parents are often forced to focus all of their attention on the child with a disability. This can lead to problems with the siblings and the family should be counseled to be aware of this potential problem. There are new financial burdens, such as durable medical equipment costs that may not be funded by the insurance companies, transportation costs, loss of 1 spouse's income, extra child care costs, and many unfunded out-of-pocket expenses such as ramps for a wheelchair, alteration of bathrooms and bedrooms, and communication and computer device alterations and adaptations (**Fig. 1**).

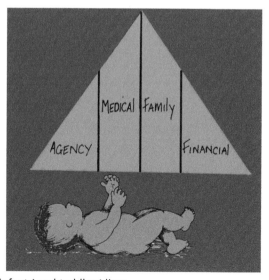

Fig. 1. Factors in infants' and toddlers' lives.

As the child ages and is in the primary school years, the family is faced with the same concerns as other typically developing families, as well as their own unique problems. What will their child do for leisure and recreation? How will they access technology? What are the mobility options available to their children? How will physical therapy affect their mobility and their quality of life? Is more physical, occupational, and speech therapy better? Why can they not have all of therapies for 1 hour, 5 days a week? Does their child need braces? What about a power wheelchair? How will they transport the wheelchair and is their home accessible?

What is the best educational plan for their children? How will they craft their child's Individualized Educational Plan (IEP) to ensure that their child gets all that they need to succeed in school? Finally, the typical social relationships between children are usually affected by their child's disability. While others are getting together for play groups, birthday parties, Little League, and soccer, families of children with disabilities often have to make choices between having more therapy or actually letting the child and the family rest from all of the other extra demands from school and therapy (**Fig. 2**).

MODELS OF MEDICAL CARE FOR CHILDREN WITH DISABILITIES

The health care provider can have a great impact on the situation depending on their approach to the family. Parents want their health care providers to provide them with information, or at least point them in the right direction to obtain the

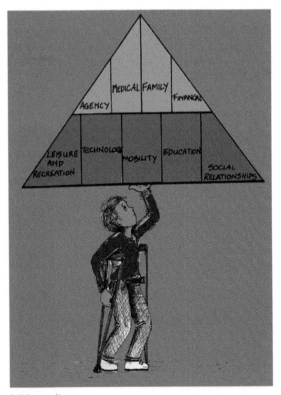

Fig. 2. Factors in children's lives.

information. They want the provider's expertise, empathy and respect, and, above all, they want to form a partnership with the provider to make decisions together to improve the life of their child and, therefore, their family. This does put some pressure on the health care professional to have the education and constant upgrading of their knowledge to best serve these families. The establishment of a partnership with the family can be a challenge at times because there are differences in style and needs, with some who are eager to be partners and others who may simply want to be told what to do.

This type of health care provision is called *paternalism*. This is the old-school method with the physician acting in the dominant and autonomous role as the arbiter of all knowledge. In this model, the patient and the parents are passive and dependent. Many of the older practitioners are only comfortable in this role.

Mutuality occurs when each participant has a unique role and responsibility. The relationship is consensual and there is a willingness to negotiate. This model is based on mutual respect and an acknowledgment of the different experience and understanding of each participant, as well as an expectation that each participant will benefit from the clinical interaction.

Family-centered care is the model toward which we should all aspire as clinicians. The Institute for Patient- and Family-Centered Care was formed in 1992 to investigate and promulgate the notion that families play a vital role in the provision of health care and well being of patients and families. The principles of family-centered care are:

- Recognizing the family as a constant in the child's life;
- Facilitating parent–professional collaborations at all levels of health care;
- Honoring the racial, ethnic, cultural, and socioeconomic diversity of families;
- Recognizing family strengths and individuality and respecting different methods of coping;
- Sharing complete and unbiased information with families on a continuous basis;
- Encouraging and facilitating family-to-family support and networking;
- Responding to child and family developmental needs as part of health care practices;
- Adopting policies and practices that provide families with emotional and financial support; and
- Designing health care that is flexible, culturally competent, and responsive to family needs.[11]

There are hundreds of articles extoling the benefits of this methodology of care delivery, but it requires a consistent effort to reach out to families to encourage their essential participation, an investment of money by the hosting organization, and an investment of time and commitment of the care providers to ensure that these principles are met.[12,13] Glenn and colleagues[14] demonstrated that the strength of the family really determined the stress of the mother. If there is a cohesive family unit, then there is an improvement in the parent feeling more in control and less stressed.

TEAM STRUCTURES FOR CARING FOR A CHILD WITH A DISABILITY

One of the largest stressors for a parent is the number of appointments that they and their child has to attend. One could list almost all of the specialties in a pediatric hospital and the family may need to see 3 or 4 of them throughout the year. This is hard enough if the family is of more than moderate means and lives near the medical center or hospital, but can be a huge problem if the patient has problems with transportation and lives further away. The parent, and often the entire family, must spend hours traveling and waiting to see the physicians and therapists.

This method of seeing many different doctors on different days and often in different locales is often the standard of care for most patients. It is very efficient for the physician, because the patient comes to them. However, they may or may not have an office that is readily accessible and they may or may not have additional resources (nursing, social work, therapists, etc). With the advent of the electronic medical record, each of the specialists can read the note of the others and get a relatively good picture of what's going on with the patient. This is the least efficient method for the family as they usually have to come in on different days.

In a *multidisciplinary* clinic, all of the specialties are centrally located, perhaps not co-located, but in close enough proximity so that the patients and family can see all of the physicians and providers in the same day. This requires a lot of care coordination and would not really be possible without the electronic medical record. Families do enjoy seeing all the people they need to see on 1 day, but if one of the services is delayed or running late, then the rest of the clinics' schedules are thrown off and the family feels anxious. There can be confusion or conflicting opinion regarding treatment plans and options, and this is difficult for families as well.

Another model is *interdisciplinary*, where there are multiple disciplines together at the same time. Many spina bifida and muscle disease clinics use the model with the neurologist, the physiatrist, an orthopedic surgeon, and occasionally the urologist. There is usually a care coordinator with nursing staff and all of the other necessary services. Typically, the care coordinator, either in concert with each of the specialists or by reviewing the chart, develops a treatment plan based on recommendations from all of the specialties. This is among the most efficient clinics for the families because they only have to come once; however, the parents and the child can become very fatigued at the end of the day after repeated recitations of their story and examination of the patient. This is the maximally inefficient clinic for the physicians because the logistics of working around all of the specialties does not permit them to see as many patients at they would in the more traditional model.

Transdisciplinary models occur at places where 1 or 2 physicians perform the roles of several disciplines. For example, a physiatrist may have the skills to diagnose and treat various neurologic disorders, can handle the medication refills, can treat movement disorders, can order equipment and therapy, and can screen for surgical indications. There is a lot of efficiency in this model, but it does put the stress on the provider and takes the other specialties "off the hook." Families often enjoy this type of care, but if the provider is not present, there is little knowledge of the patient in the system.

Regardless of the model utilized in the care of these patients, the basis for true collaborative care and effective treatment is good communication.

BASIC STRUCTURE FOR DIALOGUE WITH THE PATIENT AND THEIR FAMILY

- *Greeting*: Do not ignore the child. Establish a connection by touching; attempt to make eye contact. Notice details about what the child is wearing or what is on their wheelchair. Acknowledge the parents and the extended family—often there are grandparents, other children, and other health care providers such as nurses or therapists.
- *Prepare for Listening*: Sit down. Look relaxed. Do not stand throughout the examination; use a chair to get to the eye level of the patient. Many children will have a communication board or device. Acquaint yourself with the patient's mode of communication.

- *Questioning*: Use closed questions (yes/no; when did a procedure occur, what medications the patient is taking) for the medical history. Use open-ended questions when possible ("What is your biggest concern right now?").
- *Effective Listening* is the first component of supporting the parents: Let the parent speak. Allow them to "tell their story." This lets the parents feel known and understood. It gives them the opportunity for catharsis, insight, and perspective. It permits them to convey the life context of the illness, its meaning and interpretation, and voices their expectations of care.

Ten ways to listen better.
1. Let the parent talk.
2. Probe the hints that the parent drops.
3. Offer facilitating remarks.
4. Ask open-ended questions.
5. Be reflective; the clinician does not have to know the answer to every problem.
6. Check for accuracy.
7. Determine the parents' expectation for treatment.
8. Practice legitimizing.
9. Maintain eye contact.
10. Ask "What else is on your mind?" before leaving the room. This can lead to a longer appointment than expected, but often helps to clarify and prioritize the patient's and family's needs.

SPECIFIC PROBLEMS OF A CHILD WITH A DISABILITY
Feeding and Nutrition

Physical growth is one of the primary measures of health and well-being in children. Abnormal growth may be a sign of disruption in a child's nutrition, environment, or health[15] Decreased body fat and growth have been associated with increased health care utilization and decreased participation in society.[16,17]

It seems intuitive to mention how important proper nutrition is to all aspects of a healthy life: Growth, muscle strength, respiratory function, cardiac function, neurologic function in a child who is already neurologically compromised, immune function, and wound healing, just to mention a few consideration. Malnutrition decreases the energy for discretionary activity, which is necessary for social interaction and school participation.[18] Proper nutrition is also important for bone growth and health. Children with poor nutrition who also take antiepileptics and other medications are often osteopenic. These patients could have osteomalacia (lack of vitamin D) or osteoporosis from disuse and poor nutrition, or probably a combination of the two. There can also be endocrine abnormalities from the initial or subsequent brain injury. This can lead to fractures, which are both painful and alter the child's ability to sit and, therefore, participate in life.[19,20]

There are many factors causing malnutrition, but the one that impacts parenting the most is actually feeding the child. Although the nutrition of able-bodied children can be difficult, it is nothing compared with the challenges that a parent of a child with dysphagia faces. These patients have prolonged feeding times (sometimes >45 minutes per meal), delayed progression of oral feeding skills, and possible respiratory disease from aspiration.[21] It seems logical to assume that, if the patient is having problems eating because of dysphagia, then the placement of a gastrostomy tube would solve those problems. However, Craig and colleagues,[22] found that the introduction of the complexity of the technology and the tubing as well as the surgery actually increased the stress of the parents. They suggested that there is a greater, not lesser need for support of these families.

Sleep Disorders

One of the most common problems that parents relate is their difficulties with their child's sleeping habits. There are many reasons for this. Sometimes it is just the fact that they child needs to be repositioned frequently, there may be a seizure disorder, or problems can be secondary to pain and muscle spasms. But often the issues are just secondary to the child's own inability to sleep through the night.[23–25] Newman and colleagues[26] found that there was a 44% chance that there was 1 sleep disorder, but there was a 23% chance that the patients would have an abnormal total sleep score, indicating more than 1 identifiable issue. They also found that there were significant problems in patients who have visual disturbances because they do not sense the normal rhythms of the day and night.

Mothers also have a 40% chance of having sleep disorders themselves as well as a similar percentage of depression.[27] Another study suggested that almost 50% of children with chronic disability have sleeping problems and this negatively affected the child, the parents, and the entire family.[28]

There are so-called sleep hygiene measures to help with sleeping. These include:

- Avoid napping.
- Avoid stimulants such as caffeine.
- Exercise if possible.
- Do not eat right before bedtime.
- Obtain adequate exposure to natural light.
- Establish a regular bedtime routine.
- Associate your bed with sleep, not watching TV or listening to the radio.

However, these measures often do not work. There are many studies in the literature on the use of melatonin, and a study by Wasdell and colleagues[29] in which there was a randomized, placebo-controlled trial of controlled release melatonin that seemed to demonstrate that this could be a helpful medication for the child and, therefore, the family.

Mental Health Challenges

There is an higher incidence of mental health and behavioral problems in children with chronic disabilities than typically developing children. However, there is a paucity of literature demonstrating this, despite significant evidence of this in most clinicians' practices. There is some literature on the effects of having a child with a disability on the mental health condition of the parents, particularly the mothers.

Thirty percent of mothers of 270 children with cerebral palsy demonstrated depressive symptoms in a study by Manuel and colleagues.[30] Nereo and colleagues[31] found that the presence of problem child behaviors in children with Duchenne muscular dystrophy led to significant stress in the mothers. He found that this was similar to those mothers of children with cerebral palsy. These were more closely related to the mother's coping with their children's behaviors than it was with the demands of physical care.[32]

Mental health issues combined with alcohol and drug abuse are a potential problem in parents of children with disabilities. The clinician must be aware of these potential problems and be willing to address them with some sort of intervention, which is usually accomplished by taking a careful history and just asking the right questions.

Getting the social workers involved early may also help to pinpoint the problem so that the family member can get professional help.

Palit and colleagues[33] presented a program in which they had parents who had older children with cerebral palsy and other disabilities counsel those parents who had younger children. This parent-to-parent interaction and support seemed to be therapeutic for both groups, if for no other reason than information was obtained and parents were less likely to feel as isolated and alone.

Cultural Influences

There is not enough room in this short article to discuss all of the differences in and the ramifications of culture on the family of a child with a disability. The family's religion, hierarchical structure, nationality, and life experiences all contribute to the manner in which members of the family respond to the diagnosis, treatment, and ongoing care of a child with a disability. It is sufficient that the clinician be cognizant of the variety of cultural differences in coping, division of labor in the home, and even religious views of disability when caring for the child and the family.[34–38]

Transition and Lifespan Issues

As the child grows older and becomes a teenager, not only are there changes secondary to growth, but many of the medical problems of childhood can worsen. For example, gastroesophageal reflux can become more troublesome and lead to increased tone. Patients can develop kidney stones from chronic dehydration. Skin problems such as ulcers are more problematic as the child gets heavier, and the skin becomes less elastic. The patient often requires orthopedic surgery for tendon lengthening, osteotomies, and, in the more involved patients, posterior spinal fusion (**Fig. 3**).

As their child ages, families are faced with many choices involving medical, social, and emotional concerns, often with little or conflicting information available to aid them in their decision making. There are huge technological advances in wheelchairs, lifts, computing and communication devices, personal computing, and do on, little of which is completely covered by insurance and requires specialized knowledge and assessment. Transportation, often obtained by purchasing a converted van, is very expensive. Most families cannot afford all of these potentially life-changing devices and assistive technology. This situation is yet another stress for families. They fear that, without the assistance these items provide, their child will be left behind and have fewer opportunities for inclusion with their peers and in their communities.

Health care providers need to be aware of all of the other arenas of a patient's life that are affected by the disability; the patient's medical problems are only a small part of their lives. Education is among the biggest concerns, and more often than not, families have to fight for all of the resources that they think will benefit their child. The development of the yearly Individualized Education Plan (IEP) often finds families in conflict with the school teachers and administrators who are trying to maximize their meager budgets while still providing appropriate services for the child with special needs. Other facets of life that typical families may take for granted, such as social relationships, leisure, and recreation, become another source of concern, and facilitating them places additional time demands on an already exhausted parent.

One of the real and growing crises in our medical system is our inability to provide adequate transition care from pediatric providers to adult providers as the patient with special needs enters adulthood. The experts in the childhood acquired chronic disabilities are pediatric specialists. There are wonderful children's hospitals throughout the world and a Shriner's system that are dedicated specifically to serving the medical

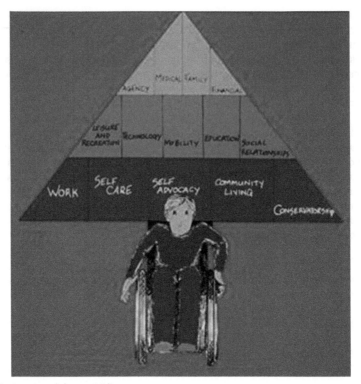

Fig. 3. Factors in adolescents' lives.

needs of children with disabilities. However, once the child turns 18, or in some cases 21, the young adult is then forced to receive services in the adult world, where many providers are unfamiliar with these disabling medical conditions, who have no experience or understanding of the diagnosis, where the treatment system is fragmented, and one in which the disabled young adult is underinsured for their needs. There are several factors contributing to this disruption in care. First, there are some pediatric specialists who are reluctant to give up their "kids," so they do not plan for the eventuality that they will become adults. The reason for this is that there is rarely a specialist or even a primary care physician who has any training or experience with childhood acquired disabilities. Most adult providers have residency and fellowship training in very different areas. For example, an adult cardiologist would likely be very uncomfortable taking care of a young adult with Down Syndrome who has had a congenital heart problem treated in infancy. Many of the surgical specialists at least have a few months of pediatric training, but it is not enough to bring any level of expertise to the complex problems of these patients. Second, another deterrent to adequate continuity of care is the fact that most children with disabilities who become adults have government-sponsored insurance. This low reimbursement model makes it very difficult for the adult provider to spend the time necessary to learn about the individual disabilities and provide the comprehensive care and services that a particular patient might need. These are the most complex patients who then as adults are often left to receive the worst care we can offer, that is, a trip to the emergency department. The uncertainty of who will provide needed ongoing medical care for their young adult son or daughter is a source of substantial stress for families. Although they have managed to keep their child alive over the years and to maximize their health status with dozens of trips to clinics and hospitals working cooperatively with the most highly trained specialists in a welcoming and family-centered children's hospital environment, their options are now drastically and devastatingly reduced. Facing the sudden reality of the need to resort to care in an emergency department because there are not physicians capable of or willing to treat their young adult children in a different setting owing to inadequate training or insurance coverage[9] can result in feelings of incredible frustration and fear regarding the future.

Once again, there are a multitude of new problems that are unique to the young adult with a disability. Most adults desire to have a job upon completion of school, and are cognizant of the many opportunities for independence, financial and otherwise, that follow. This becomes a significant challenge because factors like lack of job training, experience, employment support, and discrimination can severely limit chances for success. The unemployment rate among adults with cerebral palsy, for example, is near 75%. As the young adult is increasingly faced with choices and decisions regarding identity, independence, self-care and self-advocacy, this period of transition is likely to be a stressful time for parents, as they, like all parents, but with other complicating factors, are grappling on their own with how to "let go." Often because of the difficulty balancing issues regarding caregiving needs and promoting independence, as well as generally more limited living and working options in addition to financial concerns, families often find themselves continuing to live under on1e roof with the familiar patterns of parent–child interactions that have become less and less than ideal, healthy, and sustainable for all involved. Parents can feel chronically exhausted, financially, physically and emotionally, from the years of direct caregiving and management of needs on multiple fronts with little time for self-care and adequate rest. The kinds of living options for adults varies widely in terms of level of support (including full-time direct care in a residential setting or group home, supported living in one's own apartment or home, assisted living, or independent living with limited services) as well as geographically, based on differing state, city, and county funding sources and services. Making a move from one's family home to any one of a number of other options can be the most difficult and traumatic event in the life of the family with a special needs child. Often, families end up choosing "not to choose" for a variety of reasons, and the young adult remains at home until a crisis occurs (often because the parent is no longer able to care for them).

Partial list of medical problems seen in an adult disability clinic
- Increased pain.
- Early arthritis.
- Difficulty sitting for long periods of time with ulcer formation.
- Progression of their movement disorder.
- Mental health issues such as bipolar disorder and depression.
- Progressive loss of ambulation as the patient ages.
- Cervical and lumbar spine problems including myelopathy.
- Progressive hydrocephalus in middle ages.
- Worsening of dysphagia and ability to eat.
- Worsening dental care with dental caries and abscesses.

Finally, there is the issue of conservatorship. In most states, when the child turns 18, they are considered adults by law. This means that they have the full rights of adults and thus can independently make decisions regarding where to live, go to school, whom to marry, how to spend their money, how to make health care decisions, and to vote and legally sign a contract. Parents can find themselves caught off guard when they discover that they no longer have the right to make certain decisions for their young adult child. For instance, making medical decisions regarding treatment and direct access to physicians and medical records is limited. If the young adult does not have the intellectual capacity to make these decisions, then conservatorship can be applied for. This is a legal process in which the parents have to obtain a lawyer (there are associated costs for the parent or guardian) and the young adult has to obtain a lawyer (this is usually done by the courts with no cost to the young adult) and they must appear before a judge who will determine which, if any, rights can be limited and taken away from the young adult. This process can be scary and costly for the family, but necessary to protect some people with more significant intellectual disabilities.

CAREGIVER QUALITY OF LIFE

Caring for a child with a disability can have both positive and negative effects on parents. The goal of all caring parents is to provide the best quality of life for their child as well as to maximize their potential. Each family's situation and coping ability is different based on the type and severity of disability of their child as well as a host of other factors including their socioeconomic status, education, culture, support network, and individual personality and parenting style. Inevitably, the family functions differently, in ways that can be perceived both positively and negatively. There can be no doubt the circumstances significantly impact the quality of life of the child and the parents in this situation. Most of the studies on the impact of caregiving have revolved around the stress and depression that the parents encounter.[30,39–43] Using studies specifically aimed at evaluating depression in parents with cerebral palsy, 2 studies demonstrated poorer quality of life than that of mothers who did not have children with a disability.[44,45]

Caring for a child with cerebral palsy, for example, can negatively impact parents in terms of demands on physical health, disrupted sleep, difficulty in maintaining social relationships, pressure on marital relationships, difficulty in taking family holidays, limited freedom, limited time, a child's long-term dependence, difficulty in maintaining maternal employment, financial burden, difficulty in accessing funding from the government and insurance, and insufficient support for various services. However, there can also be positive aspects. A parent's ability to build new social networks and to have pride in dedicating one's life to their child's well-being is important, and parents can draw inspiration from their children.[46]

In the Davis and colleagues article, the authors obtained open ended statements from the family which illustrate some of the gamut of experiences parents express regarding caring for their children with disabilities. Those who had better support and perhaps had a personality which was more accepting expressed:

I think we have a really good quality of life probably because of the kind of person I am, like that I'm a happy person generally. (Mother of Molly aged 3 years, GMFCS level II)

It's good because we're well supported. And I think, you know, it doesn't surprise me that families who are less supported have issues with depression and ill-health. (Mother of Tim aged 9 years, GMFCS level V)"

I think that our quality of life is quite good… I think that we're fortunate in that she's not much more severely disabled… I'm one of those that think there's always a lot worse position than yours. (Father of Belinda aged 15 years, GMFCS level IV)

Others did consider that their quality of life was poor or nonexistent:

What quality of life? I don't have one. I really don't… I have absolutely no social contact other than the support group that is still there at Kindy. (Mother of Sarah aged 5 years, GMFCS level II)

I don't feel like I have a life a lot of the time. Everything I do revolves around him. I think it was probably worse in the early years… but these last 3¹/2 years have been really hard. (Mother of Carl aged 3 years, GMFCS level IV)

I'd say fairly stressed… There's always something that's coming up and always appointments that Cooper has to go to… so yeah look its pretty stressful. (Father of Cooper aged 9 years, GMFCS level V)

As expected, the response depended on the child's condition and age at the time of the survey:

I think our quality of life changes a lot too. I know when we have a long period of illness, I start to get really rest- less…So on the whole it's…I guess it's the same as anyone when things are going well you feel better about it. (Mother of Michelle aged 9 years, GMFCS level V)

It's not a very straightforward answer… But over the years you learn to improve your quality of life no matter what… In the beginning it was bad, really bad but at the moment it's not bad. (Mother of Stephen aged 18 years, GMFCS level V)

Raina and colleagues[7] addressed the health and wellness of caregivers of children with cerebral palsy by utilizing a model which tried to evaluate the universe surrounding the child (**Fig. 4**). In this model, the background and context included the socioeconomic status of the family. The characteristics of the child in terms of level of function and behavior are assessed. The caregiver stress is measured as caregiving demands and perception of formal care. Self-perception is an important intrapsychic factor. As with all stimuli, either positive or negative, there are coping factors: Social support, family function, and stress management. The outcomes of their assessment was psychological health of the parents as well as physical health. They demonstrated that

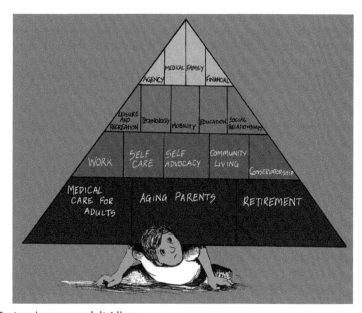

Fig. 4. Factors in young adults' lives.

their model was effective in outlining the factors, but felt that further research in all of these areas was warranted to determine what weight these factors have on the parent's quality of life. It is rather obvious that the quality of life "depends."

Brehaut and colleagues[47] demonstrated that there are self-reported physical and mental differences between parents of children with disabilities and those of able-bodied children. They also found a relationship between their socioeconomic status and the increase in these health problems. They found higher levels of distress and chronicity of distress, increased depression, increased peptic ulcers, increased migraine headaches, increased back pain, increased hypertension and heart disease, and an increased cancer rate. The authors appreciated the limitations of their study was that these were self-reported symptoms, but they were drawn from a sample of over 9000 children with disabilities in Canada.

Hayes and Watson, in a meta-analysis found that parents of children who had the diagnosis of autism spectrum disorder had a much higher stress level, even more than those of children with severe physical disabilities.[48] Although many patients with childhood disabilities also have a component of intellectual disability in addition to their physical limitations, Kishore[49] found few differences in negative and positive coping skills in children who had physical disabilities and intellectual disabilities compared with those who just have intellectual disabilities.

SUMMARY AND PERSONAL EXPERIENCES

Reid and colleagues[50] interviewed parents whose disabled children had grown up, and asked them to share lessons learned and tips for new parents of children with disabilities. The title of their article was "If I knew then what I know now." Although it is not common to have the author of an article cite personal references, I am a pediatric orthopedic surgeon who is the father of a 32-year-old young man who has total body cerebral palsy GMFCS IV, as well as dystonia and bipolar disorder. As a physician and surgeon, I also have a very large cerebral palsy practice and see a significant number of adult patients with disabilities. Our family has lived a unique journey, forever transformed by the life of our son and, therefore, we are intimately familiar with many of the issues discussed in this article. Our son has had over 20 major surgeries, requires 24/7 care, receives supported living services while living in his home near us, with a friend, who also has cerebral palsy.

So, what follows is a bit of what have I learned in my 32 years as a parent and a physician caring for patients with cerebral palsy and other disabilities:

- Parents are often focused on a cure for their child, including new and unproven treatments like hyperbaric oxygen, stem cells, and so on, but some families cannot wait for studies and evidence of efficacy. Many have been harmed physically and economically by seeking therapies that do not work.
- Simple insights have led to great changes in care. For example, the gross motor classification system allowed researchers to stratify their subjects to determine all aspects of social, epidemiologic, and treatment methodology. Being able to more completely define and recognize dystonia (as opposed to spasticity) changed the way we understood its contribution and impact on the overall functioning of the more severely involved patients, and this has changed our management, treatment, and outcomes.
- Parenting a child often means facing a series of losses and ongoing grief, and then moving forward to make adjustments. One has to change expectations about what a "normal" childhood is, having a "typical" family life, marriage, vacation, and so on. Many major milestones most parents and young adults anticipate

may come and go unachieved but not unnoticed: Walking, first date, driving, sexual and romantic relationships, advanced education, and so on.

- There is a huge disparity in health care options, treatment ,and outcomes between children and adults with disabilities.
- For all childhood disabilities, treatment is important, but prevention is the real hope.

The ying to the yang is just as important; life with a son or daughter with a disability can enrich, expand, and educate us on many levels. When a family has a child with a chronic disability, there are many opportunities to make ourselves, our families, and our communities better, like:

- Learning not to "sweat the small stuff" and distilling the essence of what really matters; prioritizing our values, and the many ways we can be more aware, sensitive, and inclusive to individual differences in our lives.
- Experiencing exhilarating joy in some of the smallest, sweetest, most unexpected things.
- Learning to stay open to possibility: Being creative and withholding judgment.

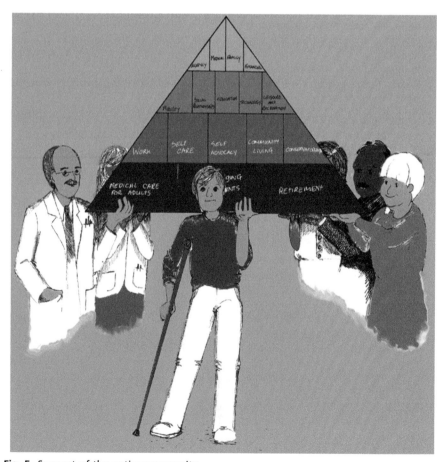

Fig. 5. Support of the entire community.

- Meeting and including in your life a wider variety of different people who can teach you a lot about yourself and the world that you are creating.
- Learning and relearning the value of compassion, patience, and a good sense of humor.
- Until recently, you got to go to the head of the line at Disneyworld.

In conclusion, the rehabilitation specialist can and should understand their role in supporting the family as well as providing care for the child. The two are intertwined. My wife developed this "Parent Wish List" which can serve as tool to help providers serve both patients and their families with respect and dignity.

I wish you would
- Treat our child as a whole person, not as parts; treat our child, not his disability.
- Look at and talk to our child.
- Notice and mention our child's abilities and strengths, not just his "deficits."
- Not judge us, we are doing the best we can.
- Not judge our child's behavior based solely on how he acts in your office; it usually does not bring out the best in him.
- Remember that we may have had to drive or ride on a bus for 6 hours for this 15-minute appointment.
- Watch your language: it is difficult to hear "impairment, deficit, abnormal, and defective" over and over again.
- Ensure that your facility and office is prepared to handle our child's physical needs.
- Imagine what life is like in our home for just 1 day.
- Respect us as partners working together with a realistic goal of health and happiness for our child and our family.

It is imperative that all health professionals work together to not only help the child and young adult, but also understand the pressures and stresses that the family incurs **(Fig. 5)**.

REFERENCES

1. Amosun SL, Ikuesan BA, Oloyede IJ. Rehabilitation of the handicapped child–what about the caregiver? P N G Med J 1995;38(3):208–14.
2. Perrin JM. Health services research for children with disabilities. Milbank Q 2002; 80(2):303–24.
3. Kelly AF, Hewson PH. Factors associated with recurrent hospitalization in chronically ill children and adolescents. J Paediatr Child Health 2000;36(1): 13–8.
4. Bromley BE, Blacher J. Parental reasons for out-of-home placement of children with severe handicaps. Ment Retard 1991;29(5):275–80.
5. Llewellyn G, Dunn P, Fante M, et al. Family factors influencing out-of-home placement decisions. J Intellect Disabil Res 1999;43(Pt 3):219–33.
6. Tong HC, Haig AJ, Nelson VS, et al. Low back pain in adult female caregivers of children with physical disabilities. Arch Pediatr Adolesc Med 2003;157(11): 1128–33.
7. Raina P, O'Donnell M, Rosenbaum P, et al. The health and well-being of caregivers of children with cerebral palsy. Pediatrics 2005;115(6):e626–36.
8. Murphy NA, Christian B, Caplin DA, et al. The health of caregivers for children with disabilities: caregiver perspectives. Child Care Health Dev 2007;33(2): 180–7.

9. Antonak RF, Livneh H. A hierarchy of reactions to disability. Int J Rehabil Res 1991;14(1):13–24.

10. Dagenais L, Hall H, Majnemer A, et al. Communicating a diagnosis of cerebral palsy: caregiver satisfaction and stress. Pediatr Neurol 2006;35(6):408–14.

11. MacKean GL, Thurston WE, Scott CM. Bridging the divide between families and health professionals' perspectives on family-centred care. Health Expect 2005; 8(1):74–85.

12. Jolley J, Shields L. The evolution of family-centered care. J Pediatr Nurs 2009; 24(2):164–70.

13. Bamm EL, Rosenbaum P. Family-centered theory: origins, development, barriers, and supports to implementation in rehabilitation medicine. Arch Phys Med Rehabil 2008;89(8):1618–24.

14. Glenn S, Cunningham C, Poole H, et al. Maternal parenting stress and its correlates in families with a young child with cerebral palsy. Child Care Health Dev 2009;35(1):71–8.

15. Samson-Fang L, Stevenson RD. Linear growth velocity in children with cerebral palsy. Dev Med Child Neurol 1998;40(10):689–92.

16. Samson-Fang L, Fung E, Stallings VA, et al. Relationship of nutritional status to health and societal participation in children with cerebral palsy. J Pediatr 2002; 141(5):637–43.

17. Stevenson RD, Conaway M, Chumlea WC, et al. Growth and health in children with moderate-to-severe cerebral palsy. Pediatrics 2006;118(3):1010–8.

18. Kuperminc MN, Stevenson RD. Growth and nutrition disorders in children with cerebral palsy. Dev Disabil Res Rev 2008;14(2):137–46.

19. Henderson RC, Lark RK, Gurka MJ, et al. Bone density and metabolism in children and adolescents with moderate to severe cerebral palsy. Pediatrics 2002; 110(1 Pt 1):e5.

20. Stevenson RD, Conaway M, Barrington JW, et al. Fracture rate in children with cerebral palsy. Pediatr Rehabil 2006;9(4):396–403.

21. Arvedson JC. Feeding children with cerebral palsy and swallowing difficulties. Eur J Clin Nutr 2013;67(Suppl 2):S9–12.

22. Craig GM, Scambler G, Spitz L. Why parents of children with neurodevelopmental disabilities requiring gastrostomy feeding need more support. Dev Med Child Neurol 2003;45(3):183–8.

23. Breau LM, Camfield CS. Pain disrupts sleep in children and youth with intellectual and developmental disabilities. Res Dev Disabil 2011;32(6):2829–40.

24. Morelius E, Hemmingsson H. Parents of children with physical disabilities - perceived health in parents related to the child's sleep problems and need for attention at night. Child Care Health Dev 2014;40(3):412–8.

25. Sandella DE, O'Brien LM, Shank LK, et al. Sleep and quality of life in children with cerebral palsy. Sleep Med 2011;12(3):252–6.

26. Newman CJ, O'Regan M, Hensey O. Sleep disorders in children with cerebral palsy. Dev Med Child Neurol 2006;48(7):564–8.

27. Wayte S, et al. Sleep problems in children with cerebral palsy and their relationship with maternal sleep and depression. Acta Paediatr 2012;101(6): 618–23.

28. Hemmingsson H, Stenhammar AM, Paulsson K. Sleep problems and the need for parental night-time attention in children with physical disabilities. Child Care Health Dev 2009;35(1):89–95.

29. Wasdell MB, Jan JE, Bomben MM, et al. A randomized, placebo-controlled trial of controlled release melatonin treatment of delayed sleep phase syndrome and

impaired sleep maintenance in children with neurodevelopmental disabilities. J Pineal Res 2008;44(1):57–64.

30. Manuel J, Naughton MJ, Balkrishnan R, et al. Stress and adaptation in mothers of children with cerebral palsy. J Pediatr Psychol 2003;28(3):197–201.

31. Nereo NE, Fee RJ, Hinton VJ. Parental stress in mothers of boys with Duchene muscular dystrophy. J Pediatr Psychol 2003;28(7):473–84.

32. Ketelaar M, Volman MJ, Gorter JW, et al. Stress in parents of children with cerebral palsy: what sources of stress are we talking about? Child Care Health Dev 2008;34(6):825–9.

33. Palit A, Chatterjee AK. Parent-to-parent counseling - a gateway for developing positive mental health for the parents of children that have cerebral palsy with multiple disabilities. Int J Rehabil Res 2006;29(4):281–8.

34. Lindsay S, King G, Klassen AF, et al. Working with immigrant families raising a child with a disability: challenges and recommendations for healthcare and community service providers. Disabil Rehabil 2012;34(23):2007–17.

35. Kaur-Bola K, Randhawa G. Role of Islamic religious and cultural beliefs regarding intellectual impairment and service use: a South Asian parental perspective. Commun Med 2012;9(3):241–51.

36. Lobato D, Kao B, Plante W, et al. Psychological and school functioning of Latino siblings of children with intellectual disability. J Child Psychol Psychiatry 2011; 52(6):696–703.

37. Huang YP, Kellett UM, St John W. Cerebral palsy: experiences of mothers after learning their child's diagnosis. J Adv Nurs 2010;66(6):1213–21.

38. Scheidegger G, Lovelock L, Kinebanian A. The daily lives and occupations of Tibetan families who have a child with disabilities. Scand J Occup Ther 2010; 17(4):286–98.

39. Park MS, Chung CY, Lee KM, et al. Parenting stress in parents of children with cerebral palsy and its association with physical function. J Pediatr Orthop B 2012;21(5):452–6.

40. Parkes J, Chung CY, Lee KM, et al. Parenting stress and children with cerebral palsy: a European cross-sectional survey. Dev Med Child Neurol 2011;53(9):815–21.

41. Pelchat D, Levert MJ, Bourgeois-Guerin V. How do mothers and fathers who have a child with a disability describe their adaptation/transformation process? J Child Health Care 2009;13(3):239–59.

42. Piskur B, Beurskens AJ, Jongmans MJ, et al. Parents' actions, challenges, and needs while enabling participation of children with a physical disability: a scoping review. BMC Pediatr 2012;12:177.

43. Sheeran T, Marvin RS, Pianta RC. Mothers' resolution of their child's diagnosis and self-reported measures of parenting stress, marital relations, and social support. J Pediatr Psychol 1997;22(2):197–212.

44. Yilmaz H, Erkin G, Nalbant L. Depression and anxiety levels in mothers of children with cerebral palsy: a controlled study. Eur J Phys Rehabil Med 2013;49(6):823–7.

45. Sajedi F, Alizad V, Malekkhosravi G, et al. Depression in mothers of children with cerebral palsy and its relation to severity and type of cerebral palsy. Acta Med Iran 2010;48(4):250–4.

46. Davis E, Shelly A, Waters E, et al. The impact of caring for a child with cerebral palsy: quality of life for mothers and fathers. Child Care Health Dev 2010;36(1): 63–73.

47. Brehaut JC, Kohen DE, Garner RE, et al. Health among caregivers of children with health problems: findings from a Canadian population-based study. Am J Public Health 2009;99(7):1254–62.

48. Hayes SA, Watson SL. The impact of parenting stress: a meta-analysis of studies comparing the experience of parenting stress in parents of children with and without autism spectrum disorder. J Autism Dev Disord 2013;43(3):629–42.

49. Kishore MT. Disability impact and coping in mothers of children with intellectual disabilities and multiple disabilities. J Intellect Disabil 2011;15(4):241–51.

50. Reid A, Imrie H, Brouwer E, et al. "If I knew then what I know now": parents' reflections on raising a child with cerebral palsy. Phys Occup Ther Pediatr 2011; 31(2):169–83.

Common Complications of Pediatric Neuromuscular Disorders

Andrew J. Skalsky, MD*, Pritha B. Dalal, MD

KEYWORDS

- Pediatric neuromuscular disorder • Nutrition • Constipation • Scoliosis
- Hip dysplasia • Sleep

KEY POINTS

- Children with pediatric neuromuscular disorders suffer from common complications.
- The complications are related to immobility and weakness.
- Scoliosis, hip dysplasia, and osteoporosis are common musculoskeletal complications.
- Constipation, gastroesophageal reflux, obesity, and malnutrition are common gastrointestinal complications.
- Disordered sleep affects both the children and their caregivers.
- Screening for these common complications can lead to healthier children with pediatric neuromuscular disorders and a resulting higher quality of life.

INTRODUCTION

Nature of the Problem

There are several pediatric neuromuscular disorders (pNMDs), such as cerebral palsy (CP), myelomeningocele, spinal cord injury, chromosomal abnormality, acquired brain injury, acquired and hereditary neuropathy, myopathy, and motor neuron disorders that all share common complications. Immobility and weakness are the primary etiologies for most of these commonly seen conditions. Musculoskeletal complications in pNMDs include hip dysplasia with associated hip subluxation or dislocation, neuromuscular scoliosis, and osteoporosis and resulting fractures. Constipation and gastroesophageal reflux (GER), along with obesity and malnutrition, are commonly

Disclosure: The authors have nothing to disclose.
Division of Pediatric Rehabilitation Medicine, Department of Pediatrics, Rady Children's Hospital San Diego, University of California San Diego, 3020 Children's Way, San Diego, CA, USA
* Corresponding author. Division of Pediatric Rehabilitation Medicine, Department of Pediatrics, Rady Children's Hospital San Diego, University of California San Diego, 3020 Children's Way, MC 5096, San Diego, CA 92123.
E-mail address: askalsky@rchsd.org

Phys Med Rehabil Clin N Am 26 (2015) 21–28
http://dx.doi.org/10.1016/j.pmr.2014.09.009
1047-9651/15/$ – see front matter © 2015 Elsevier Inc. All rights reserved.

pmr.theclinics.com

experienced gastrointestinal (GI)-related complications. Disordered sleep also is frequently observed, and this affects not only the patients but also caregivers.

MUSCULOSKELETAL COMPLICATIONS

Musculoskeletal complications, such as limb contractures, hip dislocation or subluxation, and scoliosis are common in pNMDs (**Table 1**). They contribute to increased disability due to decreased motor performance, mobility limitations, reduced functional range of motion, loss of function for activities of daily living (ADLs), decreased quality of life (QOL), and increased pain.

Scoliosis in pNMDs leads to multiple problems, including poor sitting balance, difficulty with upright seating and positioning, pain, and preclusion of the ability to sit upright in a wheelchair.[1] Screening for spinal deformities is important because it can have several clinical implications. Unfortunately, spinal deformity is neither preventable nor responsive to nonsurgical modalities such as bracing. Unlike idiopathic scoliosis, neuromuscular scoliosis almost always progresses. Early detection and screening are crucial for proper and ideal management of scoliosis.

The Adam forward-bend test is the primary screening test for neuromuscular scoliosis and should be performed on all patients with pNMDs. The screening examination is performed by having the patient bend forward as far as possible, flexing the cervical and thoracolumbar spine. If a patient is unable to stand, this can be performed in the seated position. Some patients will require postural support if they are unable to sit independently. The patient is viewed from behind focusing on the rib cage. The examiner is looking for one side of the rib cage to be higher than the other next to the vertebral column. The convex side of the scoliosis is the side with the rib hump. In obese patients, smaller curves can be missed, especially in the lower lumbosacral spine.

If a spine curve is detected or the patient's body habitus precludes the test's sensitivity, spinal radiographs should be performed. Anteroposterior (AP) and lateral spinal radiographs with the patient either sitting or standing, based on the individual's function, are generally sufficient. On the AP film, the Cobb angle is measured.[2] Serial measurements should be performed using the same anatomic landmarks to ensure comparable measurements (**Fig. 1**).

Hip subluxation and dislocation due to hip dysplasia are frequently encountered in children with pNMDs. Hip dysplasia is a condition of the hip that may be present at or shortly after birth with inadequate acetabular formation. At birth, neonates have a shallow acetabulum. As they grow, the acetabulum usually deepens and contours around the femoral head. When infants have decreased muscle tone, strength, and movement, the acetabulum remains shallow due to the reduced force applied to the acetabulum by the femoral head. Hip dysplasia is most commonly seen in pNMDs

Table 1						
Incidence of musculoskeletal complications of pediatric neuromuscular disorders						
Musculoskeletal Complications	Cerebral Palsy	Myelomeningocele	Duchenne Muscular Dystrophy	Spinal Cord Injury	Charcot-Marie-Tooth	Spinal Muscular Atrophy
Scoliosis, %	38–64	20–94	63–90	100[a]	10	70–100
Hip dysplasia, %	2–60	1–28	35	29–82	6–8	11–38

[a] If injured before adolescent growth spurt.

Adapted from Driscoll SW, Skinner J. Musculoskeletal complications of neuromuscular disease in children. [review]. Phys Med Rehabil Clin N Am 2008;19(1):163–94. PMID:18194756.

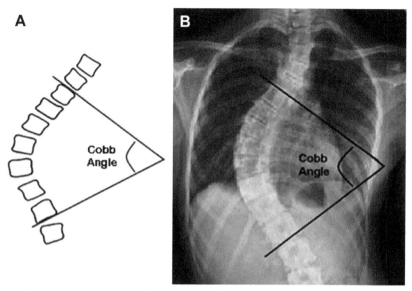

Fig. 1. Measurement of the Cobb Angle on (*A*) animated diagram and (*B*) AP spine radiograph.

with congenital or early-onset paresis, such as myelomeningocele, CP, congenital my-opathies, congenital muscular dystrophies, and spinal muscular atrophy types 1 and 2. The presence of hip dysplasia predisposes children with pNMDs to progress toward hip subluxation and eventually dislocation. The primary physical examination maneuver screening for hip subluxation or dislocation is the Galeazzi sign or Allis sign. The maneuver is performed by laying the patient supine, flexing the hips and knees, and examining the knee heights. If the knees are not at the same level, the test is positive. The pathologic side is the lower knee height and subluxation is often associated with decreased hip abduction range of motion (**Fig. 2**). In the setting of complete dislocation, hip abduction can be reduced, normal, or excessive. If the Galeazzi sign is positive, an AP radiograph of the pelvis should be obtained.

In addition to joint complications, bone health also is significantly affected in pNMDs. There are several factors contributing to poor bone health in pNMDs, such as decreased mobility, muscle weakness, and medication side effects, such as gluco-corticoid treatment for Duchenne muscular dystrophy (DMD). The consequences of osteoporosis in pNMDs can be long-bone fractures and vertebral compression

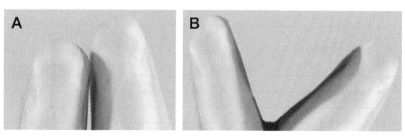

Fig. 2. Galeazzi or Allis sign (*A*) suggestive of right hip dislocation and (*B*) associated decreased abduction range of motion.

fractures that can result in bone pain and a reduced QOL. Fractures can occur with minimal trauma, such as during transfers or with rotation, such as forearm supination to start a peripheral intravenous line. Osteoporosis is more severe in nonambulatory children with pNMDs. Sufficient vitamin D levels are required for normal skeletal development and mineralization. A recent study found that 97% of children with myelomeningocele had vitamin D levels in the insufficient range (<30 ng/mL) and 48.5% had levels less than 10 ng/mL. There was a significant correlation between serum 25-hydroxyvitamin D (25[OH]D) and osteoporosis, concluding that vitamin D supplementation may be helpful.[3] There is insufficient evidence that weight-bearing activities are an effective intervention to improve bone density; however, there is also inadequate evidence to support the use of vitamin D supplementation to decrease fractures.[4] A general rule is to supplement with double the recommended dietary allowance amount for age (Table 2). Serum levels of 25(OH)D should be screened in late winter, as levels reach their nadir in the northern hemisphere due to shortened daylight and the supplemental vitamin D3 (cholecalciferol) dose should be adjusted accordingly to achieve the desired level.

Pediatric neuromuscular disorders are associated with a number of associated musculoskeletal complications. Careful screening can lead to earlier detection. Detection often results in proactive responses, which may limit the progression of the complications and reduce the negative impact on QOL.

GASTROINTESTINAL COMPLICATIONS

Several factors contribute to GI complications in pNMDs. Constipation, GER, and dependence for feeding can lead to malnutrition. Conversely, obesity can result due to decreased caloric needs.

Constipation is almost invariable in children with mobility impairment. The reliance on a wheelchair for mobility increases the risk of constipation. More than 50% of children with severe generalized CP[5] and almost half of boys with DMD experience constipation after transitioning to full-time wheelchair use.[6] The decreased physical movement and reduced time upright results in a slower GI transit time. This results in increased time in the colon for water absorption, which results in hard, dry stool. The Bristol scale has been developed to communicate stool texture and assess constipation.[7]

Prescription or over-the-counter medications are often necessary to prevent or minimize the symptoms of constipation. Polyethylene glycol 3350 (PEG 3350) is a colorless, odorless, and nearly tasteless compound that can be added to most fluids to help regulate constipation associated with immobility. The primary mode of action is thought to be through the osmotic effect of polyethylene glycol 3350, which causes water to be retained in the colon and limits the increased reabsorption of fluid due to the decreased transit time. Because PEG 3350 prevents the formation of hard stool,

Table 2 Vitamin D3 (cholecalciferol) dosing		
Age	RDA Dose, IU	Starting Dose, IU
0–6 mo	200	400
7–12 mo	260	500
1–8 y	1000	2000
9–18 y	1300	2500

Abbreviation: RDA, recommended dietary allowance.

it is better used for prophylaxis, as opposed to treatment of already present severe constipation. Stimulants, such as bisacodyl or enemas, can be necessary if a patient has acute constipation or fecal impaction. Adequate fluid intake is necessary to minimize constipation. Dietary fiber supplementation may be a useful, but requires adequate hydration to ensure a softer stool texture. Inadequate hydration along with fiber supplementation can result in large amounts of hard stool.

The most ideal nutrition management and caloric needs of children with pNMDs is not known. Poor nutrition in pNMDs is of 2 spectrums: hypoalimentation and hyperalimentation. Causes of hypoalimentation are multifactorial, including severe dysphagia, gastroesophageal dysmotility, delayed gastric emptying, prolonged meal time due to neuromuscular weakness, and dependent feeding. Hyperalimentation is caused by decreased caloric needs due to decreased mobility without associated modifications to diet, guilt on behalf of caregivers resulting in lack of caloric restraints, abundant access to high-caloric foods, and medications resulting in appetite stimulation, such as corticosteroids for the treatment of DMD.

Increased body fat percentage as well as decreased lean tissue mass in individuals with pNMDs in comparison with anthropometrically similar controls has been confirmed by multiple investigators.[8–13] Age, height, weight, and body mass index (BMI) are often used to estimate caloric needs in the general population. BMI is not an appropriate index in neuromuscular disorders because it greatly underestimates the amount of fat mass in comparison with the general population.[11,12] Most equations using anthropometrics to estimate caloric need are based on able-bodied subjects. Using the same information to estimate caloric needs in pNMDs results in an overestimation of calories. Similarly, clinicians strictly relying on the appearance of an individual with pNMDs to estimate caloric needs is problematic. Given the increased body fat in pNMDs, a low BMI may still represent a body composition with increased body fat percentage. For example, based on the dual-energy X-ray absorptiometry data from the author's previous publications, to achieve a similar body fat percentage as a 10-year-old able-bodied boy at the 50th percentile weight-for-age, a boy with DMD would be below the 10th percentile weight-for-age.

The authors of the consensus statement for standard of care in spinal muscular atrophy (SMA) also concluded that BMI is not an adequate measure of obesity or underweight, and a normal BMI for age likely does not represent the ideal weight for children with SMA. There is altered body composition in children with SMA, and despite being significantly underweight based on standard age, weight, and height growth charts and percentiles, the children may have adequate fat mass.[14]

The resting energy expenditure (REE) in pNMDs has been measured in several studies.[15–21] The development of obesity in children with DMD is not primarily because of a low REE but because of other causes, such as a reduction in physical activity and/ or overfeeding. Similar trends have been observed in CP. Nonambulant children with CP have significantly lower total energy expenditures, which is largely due to decreased activity levels.[19–21]

Interventions are required for unintentional weight gain or loss. Metformin has been used for weight management in obese patients with pNMDs, and has shown positive effects on weight management and reduced metabolic syndrome. Metformin is dosed as low as 425 mg daily in younger children and can be increased up to 1000 mg two times daily.[22] Undesirable weight loss is often due to dysphagia; therefore, medications are not as effective. The primary intervention for malnutrition is a feeding tube, but daily supplemental shakes are often implemented before placing a feeding tube.

Individuals with pNMDs have different nutritional needs in comparison with the general population. Clinicians must guide patients and families to promote good nutritional management to prevent malnutrition and obesity. The physical and psychosocial impact of nutrition and feeding on children and their families should not be overlooked. Excessive weight gain can lead to decreased functional mobility as well as increased caregiver burden. As mealtimes increase due to oropharyngeal weakness, less time is available for other recreational activities. The inability to self-feed can make children with pNMDs seem more dependent than their peers. It also can lead to a feeling of loss of control for patients.

DISORDERED SLEEP

Severe sleep disorders are present in more than 75% of children with pNMDs.[23] There are many components contributing to disordered sleep, including poor initiation and poor maintenance of sleep. Neuromuscular restrictive lung disease and hypoventilation, poor bed mobility, body positioning discomfort due to scoliosis and/or contractures, adjustment to a breathing apparatus such as a bilevel positive airway pressure mask, and abnormalities of the central nervous system with resulting abnormal circadian rhythms can all disrupt sleep.[24–28]

The normal sleep cycle consists of 5 stages of sleep divided into 2 categories: rapid eye movement (REM) and non-REM sleep. Non-REM includes stages 1 to 4. Stage 1 non-REM is the initiation of sleep and generally lasts 15 to 30 minutes. Stage 2 non-REM is intermediate sleep or alpha rapid-wave sleep and accounts for approximately 50% of total sleep time. Stages 3 and 4 are restorative sleep or delta sleep and are usually 15% to 20% of total sleep time. Stage 5 REM sleep is when dreaming occurs. The stages typically cycle every 90 minutes throughout the night.

Physical treatments, such as alternating pressure mattress overlays and adjustable beds to decrease pressure, may help alleviate some of the sleep disturbances; however, medications are often needed to promote adequate sleep.

Several studies in children report that melatonin may be beneficial for sleep, but the effectiveness of melatonin depends on dose, the individual sensitivity of the patient, and the time of administration. Very few adverse effects have been reported. Conversely, one randomized controlled trial of melatonin found children gained little additional sleep on melatonin. Although they fell asleep significantly faster, their waking times became earlier.[29]

It is generally accepted that efforts should be made to avoid antihistamines and benzodiazepines for long-term sleep management and should be limited to only intermittent use. Although they may increase total sleep time, the effects are generally due to increases in stage 2 sleep but decreases in stages 3 and 4. There is also a development of tolerance to the sedation side effects, which renders the medications less effective over time.

An alternative approach is to use the side effects of commonly prescribed medications, such as baclofen dosed nightly. The sedation side effect can be more pronounced when dosed only nightly. Neither baclofen nor tizanidine interupt the normal stages of sleep while still providing some degree of sedation to aid in both sleep initiation as well as sleep maintenance. In addition, the antispasmodic effects can reduce tone and discomfort contributing to improved sleep maintenance.

Sleep disturbance is a common problem in children with pNMDs. Effective physical and pharmacologic treatments are needed to ameliorate the sleep problems. Melatonin is the most assessed and safest pharmaceutical choice for pNMDs, but trazodone and mirtazapine are also widely used and appear to be effective. Both trazodone and mirtazapine are labeled as antidepressants, they both contribute to improved sleep initiation and maintenance without disrupting the restorative stages of sleep and are generally safe and well tolerated.[30]

SUMMARY

There are several common complications associated with pNMDs, primarily influenced by decreased mobility. Scoliosis, hip dysplasia, osteoporosis, constipation, nutrition, and sleep are frequently problematic. Early detection and/or addressing these issues should lead to healthier children living with pediatric neuromuscular disorders and a resulting higher QOL not only for the patients but also their caregivers.

REFERENCES

1. Hart DA, McDonald CM. Spinal deformity in progressive neuromuscular disease: natural history and management. Phys Med Rehabil Clin N Am 1999;9(1):213–32, viii.
2. Cobb JR. Outline for the study of scoliosis. The American Academy of Orthopedic Surgeons Instructional Course Lectures, vol. 5. Ann Arbor (MI): Edwards; 1948.
3. Okurowska-Zawada B, Kozerska A, Żelazowska B, et al. Serum 25-hydroxyvitamin D, osteocalcin, and parathormone status in children with meningomyelocele. Neuropediatrics 2012;43(6):314–9.
4. Fehlings D, Switzer L, Agarwal P, et al. Informing evidence-based clinical practice guidelines for children with cerebral palsy at risk of osteoporosis: a systematic review [review]. Dev Med Child Neurol 2012;54(2):106–16.
5. Veugelers R, Benninga MA, Calis EA, et al. Prevalence and clinical presentation of constipation in children with severe generalized cerebral palsy. Dev Med Child Neurol 2010;52(9):e216–21 PMID: 20497454.
6. Pane M, Vasta I, Messina S, et al. Feeding problems and weight gain in Duchenne muscular dystrophy. Eur J Paediatr Neurol 2006;10(5–6):231–6.
7. O'Donnell LJ, Virjee J, Heaton KW. Detection of pseudodiarrhoea by simple clinical assessment of intestinal transit rate. BMJ 1990;300(6722):439–40 PMID: 2107897.
8. McDonald CM, Carter GT, Abresch RT, et al. Body composition and water compartment measurements in boys with Duchenne muscular dystrophy. Am J Phys Med Rehabil 2005;84:483–91.
9. Forbes GB, Griggs RC, Moxley RT 3rd, et al. K-40 and dual-energy X-ray absorptiometry estimates of lean weight compared. Normals and patients with neuromuscular disease. Ann N Y Acad Sci 2000;904:111–4.
10. Pruna L, Chatelin J, Pascal-Vigneron V, et al. Regional body composition and functional impairment in patients with myotonic dystrophy. Muscle Nerve 2011; 44(4):503–8.
11. Skalsky AJ, Abresch RT, Han JJ, et al. The relationship between regional body composition and quantitative strength in facioscapulohumeral muscular dystrophy (FSHD). Neuromuscul Disord 2008;18(11):873–80.
12. Skalsky AJ, Han JJ, Abresch RT, et al. Assessment of regional body composition with dual-energy X-ray absorptiometry in Duchenne muscular dystrophy: correlation of regional lean mass and quantitative strength. Muscle Nerve 2009;39(5): 647–51.
13. Palmieri MD, Bertorini MD, Griffin JW, et al. Assessment of whole body composition with dual energy X-ray absorptiometry in Duchenne muscular dystrophy: correlation of lean body mass with muscle function. Muscle Nerve 1996;19:777–9.

14. Wang CH, Finkel RS, Bertini ES, et al, Participants of the International Conference on SMA Standard of Care. Consensus statement for standard of care in spinal muscular atrophy. J Child Neurol 2007;22(8):1027–49.

15. Gonzalez-Bermejo J, Lofaso F, Falaize L, et al. Resting energy expenditure in Duchenne patients using home mechanical ventilation. Eur Respir J 2005; 25(4):682–7.

16. Shimizu-Fujiwara M, Komaki H, Nakagawa E, et al. Decreased resting energy expenditure in patients with Duchenne muscular dystrophy. Brain Dev 2012; 34(3):206–12.

17. Zanardi MC, Tagliabue A, Orcesi S, et al. Body composition and energy expenditure in Duchenne muscular dystrophy. Eur J Clin Nutr 2003;57(2):273–8.

18. Hankard R, Gottrand F, Turck D, et al. Resting energy expenditure and energy substrate utilization in children with Duchenne muscular dystrophy. Pediatr Res 1996;40(1):29–33.

19. Walker J, Bell K, Boyd R, et al. Energy requirements in preschool-age children with CP. Am J Clin Nutr 2012;96:1309–15.

20. Bell KL, Samson-Fang L. Nutritional management of children with cerebral palsy. Eur J Clin Nutr 2013;67:513–6.

21. Rieken R, Goudoever J, Schierbeek H, et al. Measuring body composition and energy expenditure in children with severe neurologic impairment and intellectual disability. Am J Clin Nutr 2011;94:759–66.

22. Casteels K, Fieuws S, van Helvoirt M, et al. Metformin therapy to reduce weight gain and visceral adiposity in children and adolescents with neurogenic or myogenic motor deficit. Pediatr Diabetes 2010;11(1):61–9.

23. Wiggs L, Stores G. Severe sleep disturbance and daytime challenging behaviour in children with severe learning disabilities. J Intellect Disabil Res 1996;40: 518–28.

24. Stores G. Sleep–wake function in children with neurodevelopmental and psychiatric disorders. Semin Pediatr Neurol 2001;8:188–97.

25. Lindblom N, Heiskala H, Kaski M, et al. Neurological impairment and sleep–wake behaviour among the mentally retarded. J Sleep Res 2001;10:309–18.

26. Didden R, Korzilius H, van Aperlo B, et al. Sleep problems and daytime problem behaviours in children with intellectual disability. J Intellect Disabil Res 2002;46: 537–47.

27. Seddon PC, Khan Y. Respiratory problems in children with neurological impairment. Arch Dis Child 2003;88:75–8.

28. Jan JE, Ribary U, Wong PK, et al. Cerebral modulation of circadian sleep-wake rhythms. J Clin Neurophysiol 2011;28(2):165–9 PMID: 21399521.

29. Gringras P, Gamble C, Jones AP, et al, MENDS Study Group. Melatonin for sleep problems in children with neurodevelopmental disorders: randomised double masked placebo controlled trial. BMJ 2012;345:e6664 PMID: 23129488.

30. Hollway JA, Aman MG. Pharmacological treatment of sleep disturbance in developmental disabilities: a review of the literature [review]. Res Dev Disabil 2011; 32(3):939–62 PMID: 21296553.

Transition to Adult Care for Patients with Spina Bifida

Joan T. Le, MD[a],*, Shubhra Mukherjee, MD, FRCPC[b]

KEYWORDS

- Spina bifida • Myelomeningocele • Adult • Transition

KEY POINTS

- Individuals with spina bifida have multisystem involvement, leading to complex physically impairing conditions.
- Individuals with spina bifida are living into adulthood.
- There is a tremendous need for adult-centered care for those with spina bifida.
- There are successful outcomes in transitional adult programs for individuals with spina bifida.

INTRODUCTION

Spina bifida (SB), Latin for "split spine," is a congenital disorder that results from the incomplete closure of the neural tube caudally. Individuals affected with SB may have multisystem involvement, leading to complex physical and psychosocial conditions.

EPIDEMIOLOGY

Closure of the neural tube is typically complete by day 28 of embryologic age; at this time, some women may not be aware of their pregnancy. Incomplete closure of the neural tube caudally results in SB. SB occurs worldwide and across all ethnic backgrounds, although certain geographic and ethnic groups may be predisposed.[1] There is an increased risk in certain populations, including Irish and other northern Europeans; although the genetic link is unclear, it seems to be related to altered folate metabolism.[2] In the United States, approximately 1500 babies are born with SB

Disclosure: The authors have nothing to disclose.
[a] Division of Pediatric Rehabilitation Medicine, Department of Pediatrics, Rady Children's Hospital San Diego, University of California San Diego, 3020 Children's Way, MC 5096, San Diego, CA 92123, USA; [b] Pediatric and Adolescent Rehabilitation Medicine, Rehabilitation Institute of Chicago, Ann and Robert H. Lurie Children's Hospital of Chicago Spina Bifida Clinic, Northwestern University Feinberg School of Medicine, 345 East Superior Street, Chicago, IL 60611, USA
* Corresponding author.
E-mail address: joanle@rchsd.org

Phys Med Rehabil Clin N Am 26 (2015) 29–38
http://dx.doi.org/10.1016/j.pmr.2014.09.007
1047-9651/15/$ – see front matter © 2015 Elsevier Inc. All rights reserved.

pmr.theclinics.com

each year.[3] In the United States, Latina women have the highest prevalence of having a child born with SB in comparison with other ethnic groups.[4] The cause is unclear as to why Latina women have the highest prevalence, but it has been hypothesized that differences in dietary habits, supplement use, or social structure may play a role.[5]

The etiology of SB is multifactorial; however, some factors that may increase a woman's risk of having a child with SB include[6–9]:

- Family history of previous neural tube defect
- Folic acid deficiency
- Altered folate metabolism
- Exposures to certain medications (including valproic acid, carbamazepine, methotrexate and other folic acid antagonists, excess vitamin A, retinoic acid)
- Alcohol consumption
- Obesity
- Fever
- Maternal diabetes mellitus

Folic acid supplementation has been shown to lower the risk of having a child with SB.[10–12] In 1992, the United States Public Health Service recommended consumption of 0.4 mg of folic acid daily to women of child-bearing age to decrease the risk of neural tube defects.[13] In 1998, the US Food and Drug Administration mandated that folic acid be added to enriched grain products, such as cereals. Since the fortification of folic acid into grain products, the United States has had a 31% decrease in the prevalence of SB, from 5.04 babies affected per 10,000 births to 3.49 per 10,000 births.[3]

INTEREST IN ADULTS WITH SPINA BIFIDA

Medical and surgical advancements, such as antibiotics, ventriculoperitoneal shunts, and intermittent catheterization for the management of back closure, hydrocephalus, and neurogenic bladder respectively, have increased the survival into adulthood for patients with SB. From 75%[14] to more than 85%[15] of children born with SB survive into adulthood. With the increased longevity of children with SB new challenges arise, one of which is transitioning to adult-centered care. US Surgeon General C. Everett Koop, MD, was a strong voice for the rights of children with disabilities. In 1984, he cohosted a national conference focusing on the need for transitional care for older adolescents living with chronic childhood conditions. This conference brought the issue of health care transition onto the national radar.

Organizations such as the American Academy of Pediatrics (AAP) have published guidelines on transition of adolescent and adult care, and provision of a medical home for those affected with chronic childhood conditions, including SB.[16,17] This challenge has been recognized not only in North America but around the world, including Europe and Australia.[18,19] The First (2009) and Second (2012) World Congresses on Spina Bifida Research and Care brought together leaders in SB from more than 30 nations to share their experiences in different specialties and countries, and promote the development of new collaborative research ideas.

The Rehabilitation Act of 1973, the Individuals with Disability Education Act in 1975, and the Americans with Disability Act in 1990 improved integration and access for those with disabilities. In addition to the enhanced integration and access for those with disabilities, role models with disabilities and mentors have played a role in providing the sense of possibility and success.[20] Such an exemplar is Tatyana McFadden, 11-time medal winner in Summer and Winter Paralympics and the person behind a landmark legislation requiring public schools to provide access to sports for students with disabilities in Maryland. This law is now a model for other states.

TRANSITIONAL CARE

Multidisciplinary clinics are the standard of care for children with SB in the United States. To maximize medical and functional outcomes it is essential for physiatrists, neurosurgeons, urologists, orthopedic surgeons, and primary care physicians to communicate and collaborate.[21]

As those with SB age, unique challenges arise. The transition to adult health care has lagged behind the medical advancements that have increased survival into adulthood. Discussions on transitioning care should occur during times of relative wellness, and not during an acute medical crisis.[22] One of the greatest barriers to transitioning to adult health care was finding access to health care providers who took care of adults with special needs, in both the primary care setting and medical subspecialties.[23,24] Transition should be a gradual process and be a coordinated approach, with the adolescent/young adult taking responsibility for the direction of his or her care with familial support.[25] The recommended age for starting the discussion on transition is 14 years, as recommended by the AAP. Fourteen is also the age at which one's Individualized Education Plan for postsecondary transition planning begins. However, if the child is developmentally appropriate and can understand his or her medical condition, and can demonstrate adherence to treatment plans, the discussion on transition can begin at an earlier age.

A transition study conducted in Canada identified youths and adults with SB, cerebral palsy (CP), and acquired brain injury (ABI). The experiences and opportunities of these unique individuals and groups were studied. Although the sample size was small for the group of adults with SB (13), the study did highlight that the adults with SB, when compared with those with CP and ABI, was the most highly educated group, had the highest percentages living alone (23.1%), and had the highest percentages of those working full-time (30.8%). However, those adults with SB had the worst self-rated health of all the subgroups.[26]

In a 25-year prospective study on the outcome of those with SB in a multidisciplinary clinic, medical needs and successful outcomes were chronicled. Patients underwent shunt revisions, scoliosis surgeries, and tethered cord releases. Of those who underwent tethered cord releases, 97% had improvement or stabilization of their preoperative status. More than 80% of the young adults with SB had social continence of the bladder, with 85% of them having attended or graduated from high school or college.[14] On the other hand, a retrospective telephone study was done on a cohort of patients with SB, who were previously seen in a multidisciplinary clinic that disbanded. Three years after the clinic disbanded, no one had coordinated their care, and up to 66% of patients with SB did not have regular medical and specialty care. There was an increase in serious morbidity, including amputation and nephrectomy.[27] Transitioning care is critically important for maintaining the health of adults with SB.

INDIVIDUALS WITH SPINA BIFIDA HAVE MULTISYSTEM CONDITIONS
Primary Care

Finding a primary care provider that is knowledgable and interested in taking care of adults with special needs is a challenge. Collaboration has been made between the AAP, American Academy of Family Physicians, American College of Physicians, and the American Society of Internal Medicine in the "Consensus Statement on Health Care Transitions for Young Adult with Special Health Care Needs."[16]

Young adults have a higher prevalence of being classified as overweight or obese.[28] Adults with SB, as with able-bodied adults, require regular primary care visits with an adult-oriented physician for annual physical evaluations, routine preventive cancer screening examinations (Pap smears, breast examinations, testicular examinations), and monitoring for metabolic syndrome. Individuals with disabilities have been noted to have worse outcomes with cancers because of late detection and treatment.[29]

Neurosurgical Care

Neurosurgeons are some of the first physicians an infant with SB and family will meet after delivery/birth. In addition to the neural tube defect, the infant may have hydrocephalus or a Chiari malformation. Hydrocephalus in infancy is significantly different from hydrocephalus, which begins in adulthood. In addition to the adult causes of hydrocephalus (tumor, meningitis, hemorrhage), infants can develop hydrocephalus from abnormal brain development, which obstructs the flow of cerebrospinal fluid (CSF), and there may be multiple points of potential obstruction of the CSF.[30] Shunt failure can happen at any time, including adulthood. Up to 25% of patients with infantile hydrocephalus can have shunt failure in adulthood with nonresponding ventricles (ie, no change in the size of the patient's ventricles, but the patient has markedly increased intracranial pressure).[31] Patients with SB and hydrocephalus have increased mortality as adults, mostly due to shunt failure. As patients and families transitioned, often they were most concerned about shunt malfunction.[32]

In addition to shunt malfunctions and Chiari complications, tethered cords and syringomyelia are other potential medical complications of adolescents and young adults with SB. Tethered cord can be a delayed complication of those with SB, usually occurring during late childhood or adolescence. However, the need for untethering in adults has been documented in the literature.[33]

When a poll was taken at the 2008 meeting of the American Society of Pediatric Neurosurgeons, 52 practitioners (approximately half of the membership) reported working at a facility in which they were unable to care for patients beyond a certain age. Many of them worried about the effect the transition would have on their patients, and 36% of the pediatric neurosurgeons did not have an identified general adult neurosurgeon to whom to transfer their patients.[21] During the transition to adult care, some patients may not have an established relationship with an adult provider in neurosurgery. Therefore, physiatrists may play a pivotal role in the referral process and in providing key information to a neurosurgeon about changes in function. This coordination can assist the surgeon in deciding if or when to proceed with surgical intervention in a given patient, as shunt or tethered cord symptoms may present with less obvious findings.

Urologic Care

Urologic care is focused on the preservation of renal function and promoting urinary continence (social continence.) Neurogenic bladder complications that can occur with patients with SB include elevated detrusor leak point pressure, vesicoureteral reflux, and detrusor-external sphincter dyssynergia. Current bladder management for children with neurogenic bladder in SB emphasizes lowering the urinary storage pressure with anticholinergic medications and using clean intermittent catheterization to avoid elevated voiding pressures. With compliance in taking anticholinergic medications and performing clean intermittent catheterization, up to 92% of children demonstrated normal renal function.[34] Botulinum toxin injections have also been used on the bladder to increase capacity.

As the patient transitions to adolescence, a small study found that puberty was associated with an increase in maximum cystometric capacity, detrusor pressure, and detrusor leak point pressure, owing to prostatic growth in males or estrogenization of female urethras.[35]

Sexual counseling should be included in the adolescent/young adult clinic visit. In a survey of adolescent/young adult patients with SB, only 52% were satisfied with their sexual lives. Women with SB were 2.3 times more likely to be sexually active than men. There is a high prevalence of erectile dysfunction in men with SB.[36] When discussing sexuality with the patient, bladder and bowel concerns should be addressed, such as bladder leakage or bowel accidents during intimacy. Discussion should also include the issue of latex allergy and (latex-free) condom use.

In one study, up to two-thirds of adults with SB did not have regular urologic follow-up.[37]

In adults with neurogenic bladder in SB, there are no established guidelines for urologic surveillance. However, in the absence of urologic disorder, a baseline video urodynamics study and repeat every 2 to 3 years, annual renal ultrasonography, and annual serum creatinine level is recommended. Any change in urologic care and/or function warrants a repeat urodynamic study; consider tethered cord in the differential as well, if there is a change in bladder care/function. If there are complications, such as recurrent urinary tract infections (UTIs), pyelonephritis, stones, hematuria, abnormality on ultrasonography, unresolved vesicoureteral reflux, or progressive renal compromise, consider further evaluation with voiding cystourethrography and nuclear medicine renal function scans.[35]

In a case series, 8 patients with SB, neurogenic bladders, and chronic UTIs developed bladder malignancies.[38] There may also be an increased cancer risk with augmentation cystoplasty, with a 1.2% incidence of bladder cancer in augmented bladders in children. For these patients, an annual cystoscopy and cytologic examination of urine is recommended.[39]

In those with chronic UTIs, most interdisciplinary clinics treat with antibiotics when there are greater than 10,000 CFU/mL in association with:

1. Urine white blood cell count greater than 50 WBC/microliter of urine
2. Fever
3. Flank pain
4. Dysuria, change in urinary pattern[40]

Those who undergo bladder reconstructive surgery as children continue to have complication risks into adulthood. Risks may include stomal complications, stones, ureteric stenosis, or bladder rupture.

Orthopedic Care

Many children with SB have orthopedic complications, including club feet, dislocated hips, scoliosis, and contractures. Some of these orthopedic conditions may progress over time. Foot deformities are the most common orthopedic abnormality in children with SB. As the patient ages, calcaneovalgus deformity is commonly seen.[41] If there is a change in the foot position and neurologic status, consider tethered cord or syringomyelia. Individuals with SB are at increased risk for low bone mineral density, hence increasing their risk for fractures.[42] Overuse injuries of the shoulder were found to be more prevalent in those propelling wheelchairs than in those using crutches. Medial knee pain from valgus stress resulting from long-term abnormalities in gait may be ameliorated with forearm crutch use (First World Congress on Spina Bifida Research and Care).

Physical Medicine and Rehabilitation: Physiatry Care

Physiatrists are uniquely trained in taking care of individuals with complex, physically impairing conditions. A person's functionality is greatly affected by the level of involvement of their SB. Motor level and a history of hydrocephalus significantly affect a patient's mobility. Young adult-onset shunt failure, tethered cord, syringomyelia, neuro-orthopedic problems, obesity, and premature skeletal aging can all contribute to functional declines and loss of ambulation in this population.[33] Despite having high-quality assistive devices, adults with SB who use wheelchairs had a lower activity level, both in the home and outside the home, in comparison with those who ambulate.[43]

Physiatrists can assist in the transition process by promoting and maximizing the young adult's ability to self-care, assisting with integration to school and work, and supporting activities of interest.[44] Responsibilities for self-care may include management of bladder and bowel programs, ordering supplies, making medical appointments, arranging transportation, and participating in the meetings for one's individualized education plan. Aside from actively encouraging self-management, the physiatrist can also assist the patient in promoting self-advocacy.

Gastrointestinal Care

In individuals having neurogenic bowels, the areas mostly affected in children with SB are the large intestine, rectum, and internal and external sphincters. Encouraging social continence with a bowel program is recommended. Eighty percent of those with SB need to be utilizing some form of bowel program. Implementing routine/regular schedule, increasing liquid intake, timed bowels, disimpaction, digital stimulation, the gastrocolic reflex (it is unknown if this reflex is intact in those with SB), retrograde enemas, and taking stool softeners or bulking agents may help.[41] Surgical anterograde continence enema may be an option for those with intractable incontinence.

Cognitive and Psychological Care

Children with SB have good verbal skills, but may have learning disabilities and difficulties with problem-solving tasks, such as decision making about treatment plans,[45] which can affect self-management of care. A retrospective chart review documented that there was a delay of 2 to 5 years in self-care or autonomy of adolescents with SB.[46] One study recommended neuropsychological evaluations during key developmental transitions (during early childhood, early adolescence, and adolescence/young adulthood)[47]; however, obtaining authorizations for these evaluations may prove difficult.

As children with SB become older, self-awareness occurs. Children may become more concerned with body image. It has been found that adolescents with SB who have low body image had a propensity for depression. Those who were not socially continent had lower self-esteem.

Gender and disability may place women with disabilities at greater risk for psychosocial problems, such as depression.[48] These women are also vulnerable to physical and psychological abuse, in addition to sexual exploitation.[49]

Full-time wheelchair users had lower scores on their quality-of-life survey, yet psychological distress symptoms did not vary in comparison with other groups.[43]

For many parents with special needs children, caring for their child has been a full-time job. Some parents may feel uneasy about "letting go" as their child transitions from the pediatric health care clinic to the adult health care system.

Resources for psychological support for both patient and parents should be provided.

Women's Health

As with the general transition of care from adolescents/young adult to adult-centered care, it is a challenge to transition a young woman's health care to adult providers who are knowledgable and interested in seeing a woman with special needs. Access to Pap smears and mammograms is difficult. The importance of folic acid supplementation should be emphasized with all women of child-bearing age and their first-degree relatives (parent and siblings), and female partners of men with SB. All women of child-bearing age should take supplements of folic acid of 0.4 mg/d. Those with previous pregnancies resulting in neural tube defects should take 4 mg/d.

Young women with SB who are pregnant should be followed by a high-risk obstetrician. Pregnancy may affect bowel and bladder care as the gravid uterus progresses. Depending on the level of involvement, it is possible that the patient may not be able to feel contractions; therefore, education on other signs of labor should be discussed (eg, rupture of membranes may cause leakage).

Social, Living, and Vocational Concerns

As patients with SB become adults, the need arises for independence in life skills, self-management, housing, and employment opportunities. Executive function issues can interfere with initiation and problem solving. The Department of Vocational Rehabilitation is available at the county or state level. Individuals can be referred to local regional centers, which may have social workers or resources available for those with disabilities. The local chapter of the Spina Bifida Association is also an asset. Local support groups or sports-related organizations for challenged athletes can help with social transition.

TRANSITIONAL PROGRAM

Developing a transitional program takes a coordinated effort involving multiple departments, health care providers, and dedicated individuals. One such transitional program had the patient meet with a nurse to orient him or her regarding the transition, summarize the medical history, had the patient tour the adult care facility, transfer medical records, and undergo transition visits at the adult clinics. The health care providers at the adult facility were involved in the adult spinal cord injury program and consisted of the departments of Physical Medicine and Rehabilitation and Urology. Although there were initial reservations about the transition, 82% of the participants had a "positive experience" even though it was difficult to engage and establish rapport with a new team of providers. Patients generally appreciated being "treated like an adult." Patients and families wanted more resources on psychological services, employment and housing opportunities, obtaining adaptive equipment, and resources on nutrition and physical activities. Some concerns of patients and families included the lack of routine neurosurgical and orthopedic follow-up, and lack of effective communication.[47] A focus group for young adults with SB in Chicago showed similar results, with individuals expressing appreciation that they were "treated like an adult," were given decision-making control by the treatment team, and looked forward to the challenge of increased responsibility for their care. However, some parents expressed concerns about losing lifelong relationships with the pediatric providers and not having as much control over medical decision making.

Five key elements for a transition program were highlighted[47]:

1. Preparation
2. Flexible timing
3. Coordination of care
4. Transition clinic visits
5. Health care providers interested in taking care of adults with disabilities

SUMMARY

Individuals with SB are living into adulthood, and as they age unique challenges arise. These patients have involvement of multiple organ systems, physical impairments and disabilities, cognitive involvement, and psychosocial challenges. There is a tremendous need for transitional care for adults with SB.

RESOURCES

Centers for Disease Control and Prevention: www.cdc.gov
Spina Bifida Association: www.spinabifidaassociation.org
SB University: www.SBUniversity.org
World Congress on Spina Bifida: www.worldcongressonsb.org/
American Latex Allergy Association: latexallergyresources.org

REFERENCES

1. Northrup H, Volcik KA. Spina bifida and other neural tube defects. Curr Probl Pediatr 2000;30(10):313–32.
2. Dunlevy LP, Chitty LS, Burren KA, et al. Abnormal folate metabolism in foetuses affected by neural tube defects. Brain 2007;130(Pt 4):1043–9.
3. Centers for Disease Control and Prevention. Available at: http://www.cdc.gov/ncbddd/spinabifida/data.html. Accessed May 1, 2014.
4. Shin M, Besser LM, Siffel C, et al. Prevalence of spina bifida among children and adolescents in 10 regions in the United States. Pediatrics 2010;126:274–9.
5. Alexander MA, Matthews DJ. Pediatric rehabilitation: principles and practice. 4th edition. New York: Demos Medical; 2010. p. 199–230.
6. Czeizel A, Metneki J. Recurrence risk after neural tube defects in general counseling clinic. J Med Genet 1984;21(6):413–6.
7. Shaw GM, Todoroff K, Velie EM, et al. Maternal illness, including fever and medication use as risk factors for neural tube defects. Teratology 1998;57(1):1–7.
8. Watkins ML, Rasmussen SA, Honein MA, et al. Maternal obesity and risk for birth defects. Pediatrics 2003;111(5 Pt 2):1152–8.
9. Wide K, Winbladh B, Kallen B, et al. Major malformations in infants exposed to antiepileptic drugs in utero, with emphasis on carbamazepine and valproic acid: a nation-wide, population-based Register Study. Acta Paediatr 2004; 93(2):174–6.
10. Mosley BS, Hobbs CA, Flowers BS, et al. Folic acid and the decline in neural tube defects in Arkansas. J Ark Med Soc 2007;103(10):247–50.
11. Carmichael SL, Yang W, Shaw GM, et al. Periconceptional nutrient intakes and risks of neural tube defects in California. Birth Defects Res A Clin Mol Teratol 2010;88(8):670–8.
12. Centers for Disease Control and Prevention. CDC grand rounds: additional opportunities to prevent neural tube defects with folic acid fortification. MMWR Morb Mortal Wkly Rep 2010;59(31):980–4.

13. Centers for Disease Control and Prevention website. Available at: http://www.cdc.gov/mmwr/preview/mmwrhtml/00019479.htm. Accessed May 1, 2014.

14. Bowman RM, McLone DG, Grant JA, et al. Spina bifida outcome: a 25-year prospective. Pediatr Neurosurg 2001;34:114–20.

15. Dillon CM, Davis BE, Duguay S, et al. Longevity of patients born with myelomeningocele. Eur J Paediatr Surg 2000;10(Suppl 1):33–4.

16. American Academy of Pediatrics, American Academy of Family Physicians, American College of Physicians, American Society of Internal Medicine. A Consensus statement on health care transitions for young adults with special health care needs. Pediatrics 2002;110(6):1304–6.

17. Burke R, Liptak GS. Council on Children with Disabilities. Providing a primary care medical home for children and youth with spina bifida. Pediatrics 2011; 128:e1645–57.

18. Roebroeck MR, Jahnsen R, Carona C, et al. Adult outcomes and lifespan issues for people with childhood-onset physical disability. Dev Med Child Neurol 2009; 51(8):670–8.

19. Sawyer SM, Macnee S. Transition to adult health care for adolescents with spina bifida: research issues. Dev Disabil Res Rev 2010;16:60–5.

20. Mukherjee S. Transition to adulthood in spina bifida: changing roles and expectations. ScientificWorldJournal 2007;7:1890–5.

21. Rekate HL. The pediatric neurosurgical patient: the challenge of growing up. Semin Pediatr Neurol 2009;16:2–8.

22. Bates K, Bartoshesky L, Friedland A, et al. As the child with chronic disease grows up: transitioning adolescents with special health care needs to adult-centered health care. Del Med J 2003;75(6):217–20.

23. Scal P, Evans T, Blozis S, et al. Trends in transition from pediatric to adult health care services for young adults with chronic conditions. J Adolesc Health 1999;24:259–64.

24. Young NL, Barden WS, Mills WA, et al. Transition to adult-oriented health care: perspectives of youth and adults with complex physical disabilities. Phys Occup Ther Pediatr 2009;29(4):345–61.

25. Binks JA, Barden WS, Burke TA, et al. What do we really know about the transition to adult-centered health care? A focus on cerebral palsy and spina bifida. Arch Phys Med Rehabil 2007;88:1064–73.

26. Young NL, McCormick A, Mills W, et al. The Transition Study: a look at youth and adults with cerebral palsy, spina bifida, and acquired brain injury. Phys Occup Ther Pediatr 2006;26(4):25–45.

27. Kaufman BA, Terbrock A, Winters N, et al. Disbanding a multidisciplinary clinic: effects on the health care of myelomeningocele patients. Pediatr Neurosurg 1994;21(1):36–44.

28. Crytzer TM, Dicianno BE, Kapoor R, et al. Physical activity, exercise, and health-related measures of fitness in adults with spina bifida: a review of the literature. PM R 2013;5(12):1051–62.

29. Roetzheim RG, Chirikos TN. Breast cancer detection and outcomes in a disability beneficiary population. J Health Care Poor Underserved 2002;13(4):461–76.

30. Brodal P. The Central Nervous System: Structure and Function. 2nd edition. New York: Oxford University Press; 1998. p. 113.

31. Baskin JJ, Manwaring KH, Rekate HL. Ventricular shunt removal: the ultimate treatment of the slit ventricle syndrome. J Neurosurg 1998;88:478–84.

32. Rauen KK, Sawin KJ, Bartelt T, et al. Transitioning adolescents and young adults with a chronic health condition to adult healthcare – An Exemplar Program. Rehabil Nurs 2013;38:63–72.

33. Vinchon M, Dhellemmes P. The transition from child to adult in neurosurgery. Adv Tech Stand Neurosurg 2007;32:3–24.
34. Kasabian NG, Bauer SB, Dyro FM, et al. The prophylactic value of clean intermittent catheterization and antocholinergic medication in newborns and infants with myelodysplasia at risk of developing urinary tract deterioration. Am J Dis Child 1992;146(7):840–3.
35. Mourtzinos A, Stoffel JT. Management goals for the spina bifida neurogenic bladder: a review from infancy to adulthood. Urol Clin North Am 2010;37(4): 527–35.
36. Diamond DA, Rickwood AM, Thomas DG. Penile erections in myelomeningocele patients. Br J Urol 1986;58(4):434–5.
37. Hunt GM. Open spina bifida: outcome for a complete cohort treated unselectively and followed into adulthood. Dev Med Child Neurol 1990;32(2):108–18.
38. Austin JC, Elliott S, Cooper CS. Patients with spina bifida and bladder cancer: atypical presentation, advanced stage and poor survival. J Urol 2007;178(3 Pt 1):798–801.
39. Soergel TM, Cain MP, Misseri R, et al. Transitional cell carcinoma of the bladder following augmentation cystoplasty for the neuropathic bladder. J Urol 2004; 172(4 Pt 2):1649–51.
40. Elliott SP, Villar R, Duncan B. Bacteriuria management and urological evaluation of patients with spina bifida and neurogenic bladder: a multicenter survey. J Urol 2005;173(1):217–20.
41. Braddom RLI. Physical medicine and rehabilitation. 2nd edition. Phildelphia: W.B.Saunders Company; 2000. p. 1213–29.
42. Marreiros H, Loff C, Calado E. Osteoporosis in paediatric patients with spina bifida. J Spinal Cord Med 2012;35(1):9–21.
43. Dicianno BE, Bellin MH, Zabel AT. Spina bifida and mobility in the transition years. Am J Phys Med Rehabil 2009;88(12):1002–6.
44. Kim H, Murphy N, Kim CT, et al. Pediatric rehabilitation: 5. Transitioning teens with disabilities into adulthood. PM R 2010;2(3):S31–7.
45. Dennis M, Barnes MA. The cognitive phenotype of spina bifida meningomyelocele. Dev Disabil Res Rev 2010;16:31–9.
46. Davis BE, Shurtleff DB, Walker WO, et al. Acquisition of autonomy skills in adolescents with myelomeningocele. Dev Med Child Neurol 2006;48(4):253–8.
47. Sawin KJ, Rauen K, Bartelt T, et al. Transitioning adolescents and young adults with spina bifida to adult healthcare: initial findings from a Model Program. Rehabil Nurs 2014;17:1–9.
48. Nosek MA, Rintala DH, Young ME, et al. Sexual functioning among women with physical disabilities. Archives of Physical Med Rehabilitation 1996;77(2):107–15.
49. Hassouneh-Phillips D, McNeff E. Low sexual and body esteem and increased vulnerability to intimate partner abuse in women with physical disabilities. Sex Disabil 2005;23(4):227–40.

The Importance of Good Nutrition in Children with Cerebral Palsy

 CrossMark

Gina Rempel, MD, FRCPC, FAAP[a,b,*]

KEYWORDS

- Cerebral palsy • Malnutrition • Growth • Nutritional assessment • Enteral feeding

KEY POINTS

- In children with cerebral palsy (CP), undernutrition has significant negative consequences.
- Poor oral-feeding skills are the primary cause of inadequate nutrition in children with CP.
- Understanding the causes of poor nutrition guides nutritional intervention.
- Overcoming the challenges inherent in the physical measurement of children with CP by using heights extrapolated from segmental measures and triceps skin fold, together with weights, weight gain velocity, and monitoring these measures on appropriate growth charts, informs care providers about the need for nutritional rehabilitation and helps monitor the progress toward collaboratively established nutrition goals.
- Understanding the multidimensional aspects of oral feeding and the timing of enteral nutrition support are important elements in the nutrition rehabilitation toolkit.

INTRODUCTION
Nature of the Problem

Cerebral palsy (CP) describes "a group of persisting, nonprogressive conditions in the development of motor control that appear very early in life."[1] "The motor disorders of CP are often accompanied by disturbances of sensation, perception, cognition, communication, and behavior; by epilepsy; and by secondary musculoskeletal problems."[2] Although the primary problems associated with CP are neurodevelopmental in nature, challenges with growth and nutrition are also common in affected children.[3–5]

Disclosure: The author has no commercial affiliations or interests that might be perceived as posing a conflict or bias.
[a] Rehabilitation Centre for Children, Inc, 633 Wellington Crescent, Winnipeg, Manitoba R3M 0A8, Canada; [b] Children's Hospital, AE 303, 840 Sherbrook Street, Winnipeg, Manitoba R1A 1S1, Canada
* Rehabilitation Centre for Children, Inc, 633 Wellington Crescent, Winnipeg, Manitoba R3M 0A8, Canada.
E-mail address: grempel@hsc.mb.ca

Phys Med Rehabil Clin N Am 26 (2015) 39–56
http://dx.doi.org/10.1016/j.pmr.2014.09.001
1047-9651/15/$ – see front matter © 2015 Elsevier Inc. All rights reserved.

As a group, children with CP are smaller and more poorly nourished than their typically developing peers. These differences between affected and nonaffected children are more marked with increasing age and with the severity of the motor impairment.[6] A complex interplay of these factors and other nutritional and non-nutritional factors impacts the growth and nutritional status of children with CP.[7]

Good nutrition is the cornerstone of health and well-being for all children, whether affected by CP or not. Weight gain and growth along predicted trajectories, reassure families and care providers that a child is thriving and is healthy. The same holds true for children with CP, but in these children the measuring and monitoring of growth is fraught with challenges that must be overcome to be able to interpret nutritional adequacy.[6,8] Understanding when a child's nutritional status is faltering is important because poor nutrition has serious consequences and is potentially remediable.[9,10]

FACTORS AFFECTING NUTRITION AND GROWTH IN CHILDREN WITH CEREBRAL PALSY

The children with CP who are at the greatest risk of having significant nutritional problems are those who present with poor weight gain at a young age,[11,12] who have significant motor impairments,[13] and who have feeding and swallowing problems.[9,14,15] Other factors affecting nutrition are detailed in **Box 1**.

Nutritional Factors

Inadequate intake
The most significant factor affecting the nutritional status of children with CP is inadequate intake to meet metabolic demands.[16] In turn, food processing and swallowing problems, which affect 30% to 40% of children with CP, are the primary reasons for inadequate intake.[5,8,17] **Box 2** describes the feeding problems that are common in children with CP.

In general, children with more significant motor impairments have more challenges with oral feeding and have poorer nutritional outcomes. Even mild feeding skill deficits can have a significant impact on the quantity of food consumed. For example, children with CP who require only minor modification of their food texture or viscosity to aid in food processing and swallowing have decreased fat stores, suggesting that they have

---

Box 1
Factors affecting growth and nutrition in children with cerebral palsy

Nutritional factors:

Inadequate intake primarily related to feeding dysfunction

Increased calorie losses

Increased calorie use

Non-nutritional factors:

Age

Genetic factors

Physical factors related to the child's neurologic condition

  Neurotrophic factors

  Lack of weight bearing and mechanical stress on the long bones

Endocrine factors

Box 2
Common feeding problems in children with cerebral palsy that hamper adequate food intake

Oral motor/food-processing problems

Swallowing difficulties and airway protection problems

Positioning difficulties

Requiring assistance with feeding

Prolonged feeding times

---

inadequate energy intake.[18–20] Other factors affecting food intake are detailed in **Box 3**.

Increased losses

Children with CP can have significant calorie losses from gastroesophageal reflux (GER). GER in children with CP is in part related to foregut motility problems related to an interaction of the enteric and the central nervous system and to positioning challenges, increased intra-abdominal pressure secondary to chronic constipation, spasticity, or musculoskeletal deformity.[22] Aside from its impact on nutritional status, GER can result in esophageal inflammation and dental erosions, and can increase the risk of aspiration.[17,21]

Energy expenditure

Ambulant children with CP have similar energy expenditures to their age-matched peers, whereas those who are marginally ambulant or nonambulant have significantly lower energy expenditures. This is largely due to decreased activity levels.[16,23–25] There has been considerable debate about the influence of muscle inefficiency, spasticity, and dyskinesia on the energy requirements of children with CP.[26] These factors were once thought to increase energy expenditure; however, they may not have as large an influence as was previously thought. At the very least, the contribution of these factors to energy expenditure is subject to considerable variability among children, even when they are matched for motor abilities.[23,27]

Box 3
Other factors that may result in inadequate energy and nutrient intake

- *Sensory factors* related to the texture and taste of foods can result in the consumption of a limited repertoire of foods that may be nutritionally incomplete

- *Fatigue* before a meal or resulting from the increased effort of eating

- *Prolonged mealtimes* cause stress and fatigue in parents and children and spoil the enjoyment of the meal[21]

- *Negative feeding behaviors* related to mealtime stress or discomfort

- *Disturbances in the sensation of hunger and satiety*[7]

- *Inability to communicate nutritional needs* due to speech impediments or intellectual disabilities

- *Secondary health conditions,* such as gastroesophageal reflux and constipation,[18] cause discomfort and therefore impact oral intake

- *Dental caries and dental malocclusion* affect the quantity of food consumed

---

Energy requirements in children with CP may increase if their activity levels increase during intensive therapy sessions or if they have an increased respiratory rate and effort. Among other things, the latter can be related to upper airway obstruction or chronic chest infections.[17]

Non-nutritional Factors Affecting Growth and Nutrition in Children with Cerebral Palsy

In general, nutritional factors have a greater impact on children's weight, whereas non-nutritional factors have a larger influence on their stature.[7] Growth may be impacted by the direct effects of the negative neurotrophic factors related to the children's underlying condition or the indirect effects of immobility and lack of weight bearing.[11,28,29] Children with asymmetric involvement of CP have decreased growth and fat mass on the more affected side, even in the face of good nutritional status and typical stature for age. This supports the impact of non-nutritional, nonendocrine factors on growth in children with CP.[28] In contrast, the decline in growth with age in children with CP, even when they are well nourished,[4] and the lack of growth spurt accompanying puberty in children with severe motor impairment, speaks to the contributions of endocrine factors affecting growth. These variations in growth may be related to alterations in growth hormone and the hypothalamic pituitary axis.[30,31] The hypothalamus has an important role in modulating satiety, appetite control, and energy homeostasis and thereby influences growth and nutritional status.[7]

UNDERNUTRITION IS A REMEDIABLE CONDITION

With the increased use of enteral nutrition support has come the understanding that malnutrition is remediable and not intrinsic to CP.[6] Weight gain is generally noted early after the introduction of enteral nutrition support in children with CP, although increases in length often lag behind the improvements in weight. Growth is generally better the earlier nutrition is optimized, suggesting a critical window during which nutritional rehabilitation will have the most beneficial effect on growth.[32,33]

THE IMPORTANCE OF GOOD NUTRITION FOR CHILDREN WITH CEREBRAL PALSY
Good Nutrition Improves General Health and Participation

In any child, poor nutrition can negatively affect growth, development, and muscle strength, immune function, and wound healing.[6,7,34] There is little direct evidence of the relationship between specific health concerns and poor nutrition in children with CP, but its effects on unaffected individuals are also applicable to undernourished children with CP.[6] For example, because poor nutrition is associated with decreased muscle strength, poorly nourished children with CP may have respiratory muscle weakness and decreased coughing strength, making them vulnerable to lower respiratory tract infections.[17] Moreover, malnutrition may hamper the resolution of these infections because of decreased immune function. Furthermore, the impaired wound healing that generally accompanies malnutrition takes on special significance in children with CP who are undergoing surgical procedures.[6] In these children, delayed wound healing may negatively impact their surgical outcomes and prolong their hospital admissions.

Given the negative impact of inadequate nutrition in children in general, there has been considerable interest in determining the specific consequences of poor nutritional status in children with CP. Brooks and colleagues[10] demonstrated that poorly nourished children with CP at all levels of severity have a greater number of secondary and chronic health conditions than children who are better nourished. Similarly, researchers in the North American Growth in Cerebral Palsy Research Collaborative[15] found correlations between general health and nutritional status in children with CP.[20] They noted that not only do undernourished children with CP who have low muscle mass have poorer general health, but those with low fat reserves have increased health care utilization and decreased participation in school and family activities.[9]

Good Nutrition Improves Brain Growth and Neurodevelopmental Outcomes

Poor nutrition can negatively impact brain growth, which leads to adverse neurodevelopmental outcomes in infants.[35] Conversely, nutritional rehabilitation may have neuroprotective effects in children with a perinatal brain injury. If these children are given a diet enhanced in calories and protein early in life, they demonstrate better brain growth, which has a positive effect on their neurodevelopmental outcomes.[36] Nutritional rehabilitation also enhances motor skill development,[37] which in turn, increases a child's exploratory behavior and learning from their environment.

Good Nutrition Impacts Bone Health

Children with CP who are nonambulant are at increased risk of having bone demineralization,[38] which is compounded by inadequate nutrition, decreased exposure to sunlight, and anticonvulsant use.[39] However, in contrast to other secondary health conditions, which are worsened by underweight status, it is the children with CP who have an increased fat mass and those who are fed via gastrostomy tubes who are at greatest risk of osteopenia-related fractures.[40] This could be related to

- More rapid accrual of body fat than bone minerals
- A direct effect of the excess weight on the bone
- The impact of the fat mass itself on the bone mineral density.[40]

Good Nutritional Status Improves Survival

Good nutrition is a powerful prognosticator of survival in children with CP. At all levels of motor involvement, children with CP who are poorly nourished are at increased risk of mortality.[10,41] Overall, survivorship in children and adults with CP has increased in the past few decades, which is also the period during which use of gastrostomy tube feeding has increased.[42,43] Some have speculated that the increased survival in people affected by CP is at least in part related to a better understanding of the nutrient requirements and more aggressive management of nutrition.[43]

ASSESSMENT OF NUTRITIONAL STATUS

Health care providers can acquire valuable information about the child's nutrition by obtaining a detailed history of the primary and secondary health conditions affecting the child and specific information related to the child's feeding, as outlined in **Box 4**.

Box 4 **Information useful in understanding a child's feeding challenges**
WHO: Persons involved with feeding; differences in feeding styles
WHAT: The type, texture, viscosity, quantity, and quality of the food consumed
WHEN: The timing, frequency, and duration of meals
WHERE: The feeding environment, distractions
HOW: The feeding routine, technique, adaptive equipment, positioning

Examining the child and observing a typical meal provides valuable insight into the child's oro-motor skills, aspiration risk, nutritional status, and fat reserves and the feeding interaction and technique. Assessing the children for micronutrient deficiencies may be important if their diets are very limited in quantity and repertoire.

All of the information obtained from the history, observation, and evaluation of the child should to be assessed within the context of the child's family. Understanding the importance of feeding as a time of nurturance for the child and his or her family, regardless of the stress that mealtime may bring, helps to establish feeding goals and nutritional rehabilitation plans. These plans are often multilayered, reflecting the multidimensional nature of the task of feeding and the expertise on many levels, which different team members, including family members, bring to the table.[21]

Anthropometric Measurements in Children with Cerebral Palsy

To evaluate the nutritional status of a child, anthropometric measurements, both individually and in comparison with each other and with those of other children, are key.

Height and weight are the most basic of the anthropometric measurements. Monitoring weight is relatively easy in children with CP, especially if a wheelchair scale is available on which children can sit or can be weighed indirectly in and out of their chairs. However, the determination of height is not straightforward in children with CP, who are difficult to measure due to the presence of joint contractures, scoliosis, variations in tone, and inability to stand.

When a standing height cannot be obtained, segmental measurements that are widely accepted as valid proxies for height in children with CP can be used.[44] Accurate measurement is essential, as any errors are magnified by the equation that is needed to translate the segmental measurements into estimated lengths (**Table 1**).

Once the height is calculated from the segmental measurements, it can be used in comparison with weight and with age and can be plotted on standard growth charts. Although there are challenges in interpretation in the measurements in children with CP compared with unaffected children, the measurements nonetheless allow for trending of weight and height in individual children and can assist in identifying faltering growth over time.

Weight for height and body mass index

In typically growing children, assessing weight in relation to height is a universally accepted concept for assessing nutritional status[46]; however, in children with CP, weight for height or body mass index (BMI) calculations are of little clinical use because they lack clinical sensitivity due to the children's altered body composition and growth:

- Weight for height measures fail to identify depleted fat stores in half of children with CP[47]
- Measurement errors are magnified by the BMI calculations
- Microcephaly or macrocephaly can skew the weight for height measurements of the children.

For example, a child with a very small head may appear poorly nourished on the weight for height measurement of a standard growth chart because the typical contribution of the weight of the head to the child's overall weight is small. Examining the child and using measurements other than the standard weight for height or BMI are required in this circumstance to assess whether or not the child is adequately nourished.

Table 1
Segmental measurements of height in children with CP who are unable to stand

Measurement	Age	Equipment	Technique	Calculation[29,44,45]
KH	All ages	KH calipers	With the child sitting, the flat blade of the caliper is placed under the child's heel. With the knee and ankle joint at 90°, the top blade of the caliper is positioned 2 cm behind the patella over the femoral condyles. The KH (cm) is the distance between the blades of the caliper.	For children 12 y and younger* Estimated height = (2.69) × KH (cm) + 24.2
TL	2–12 y	Tape measure	The tibia is measured on the medial side. With the child sitting or supine, find and mark the joint space between the tibia and the femur. Then mark the distal edge of the medial malleolus. The TL is the distance between these points in centimeters.	Estimated height = 3.26 × TL (cm) + 30.8

Abbreviations: CP, cerebral palsy; KH, knee height; TL, tibial length.
* For individuals over 12 years of age refer to the tables in by Chumlea.[45]

Triceps skin fold measurement
Because weight for height and BMI do not identify children with CP who are under-nourished, other measurements to enhance the interpretation of their nutritional status are required. The clinical measurement that performs best as a screening test for depleted fat stores in children with CP is a triceps skin fold (TSF) measurement less than the 10th percentile for age as measured on standard charts.[47–49] The TSF can be easily measured without causing distress, as outlined in **Box 5**.

The TSF measurement generally underestimates the fat stores in a child with CP, in whom considerable fat is stored internally and is therefore inaccessible to fat-fold measurements.[47] This fact must be taken in to consideration during nutritional rehabil-itation. Targeting a goal TSF between the 10th and 25th percentiles and not the more usual 50th percentile for age is appropriate for children with CP because of the differ-ences in fat distribution.

Although the TSF is a valuable screening tool for fat depletion, it cannot be used in isolation to calculate overall body fat. To calculate body fat (see "Body composition" section, later in this article), indirect or direct measurements of body composition are required. However, as these are often inaccessible in clinical practice, computing the total body fat measurements using the subscapular fat fold and the TSF in CP-specific equations developed by Gurka and colleagues,[50] is a good predictor of total body fat, especially in children with CP who are ambulant.[51]

Mid-arm circumference
Interest in using mid-arm circumference (MAC) measurements in the children with malnutrition has increased recently.[34] The MAC is a measure of the child's muscle mass, and bone and fat reserves, and, therefore, like other measurements in children with CP, is affected by differences in body composition and growth compared with typical children. However, like TSF measurements, it is reproducible and can be compared with other children on the MAC chart developed either by Frisancho[48] or the World Health Organization (WHO).[49] **Box 6** illustrates an example of using the MAC and TSF measurements.

All of the anthropometric measurements (weight, height, TSF, and MAC) can be repeatedly measured and compared to monitor overall growth. Weight gain velocity between visits in grams per day helps to demonstrate weight plateaus. Expressing the growth parameters as standard deviations (z-scores) allows for comparison of actual numbers. This has an advantage over trying to gauge the trajectories on percentile charts, especially when the children plot far from the expected percentiles on standard growth charts. For example, if the weight is plotted on a standard growth chart and is always well below the third percentile, it is difficult to gauge changes over time. But if one knows that the z-score was −3.19 at the last clinic visit and now is −2.98, this is an improvement, which may not be seen on a standard percentile plot.

Box 5
Measuring a triceps skin fold (TSF)

- Identify the point halfway between the acromion and distal end of the humerus
- Using the thumb and forefinger, lift the fat overlying the triceps muscle away from the muscle
- Measure the width of the fat fold in millimeters with appropriate calipers

> **Box 6**
> **Using the mid-arm circumference (MAC) and TSF measurements in nutritional assessments**
> Using the MAC in combination with the TSF provides valuable information to share with the children's families when planning nutritional rehabilitation. For example, if a child who appears to be very lean has a TSF measurement at the 25th percentile for age but the MAC measurement is only at the 5th percentile for age, it suggests that the child has adequate calorie intake but appears very lean because of low muscle (lean body) mass. If both the MAC and the TSF are low, muscle depletion and low body fat reserves may be present.

Specialized growth charts

As mentioned previously, comparing children with CP with typically growing children on standard growth charts is fraught with challenges because of alterations in body composition and structure in children with CP. However, growth charts on which the individual weights of children with similar motor impairments can be compared has more utility. Such growth charts have been developed using a large sample of children whose information is captured in the Life Expectancy Project.[10] Brooks and colleagues developed multiple CP-specific growth charts stratified by tube feeding status and functional severity using the well-validated clinical algorithm, the Gross Motor Function Classification Scale (GMFCS).[52] The 5 GMFCS levels group children in age-bands and define trajectories of motor function over time. Children in level 1 have the best motor function and are able to walk without limitation, whereas those in level 5 have little independent mobility and are transported by others in manual wheelchairs. As there are significant differences in the children's weight and growth in relation to motor function, separate growth charts for each level provide important information about the weight of children compared with other children with a similar level of motor function. Children who are classified as GMFCS 5, are not only very different in motor function compared with children in other groups, but they are also more likely to have fragile and complex health status, grow more poorly, and require enteral nutrition support more often than children in other groups.

The CP-specific growth charts[10] describe not only the weight gain and growth characteristics of children at various levels of function, they also identify the weight-for-age percentile (20th percentile), at which point the children are at increased risk of morbidity and mortality. Thus, a single measurement can be used to provide some insight into a child's nutritional risk. This is important, because even though validated measurements appropriate for children with CP, as described previously, are available, they are still not widely applied in clinical settings.

These growth charts are population-based and will have to be validated in clinical settings. Further research also is required to see if nutritional rehabilitation will mitigate the increased risk of mortality identified in the children who plot in the "zone of concern" on the CP-specific growth charts.[46]

These charts are valuable tools in opening the discussions regarding nutritional rehabilitation with families, as parents can see how their child is fairing compared with children with similar motor challenges.[46] If a child's weight for age is consistently plotting below the 20th percentile, health care providers knowing the significance of this, at least on a population level, can reinforce the importance of improving the nutrition to avoid the morbidity and mortality risk associated with this low weight for age.

Body composition

Measures of body composition quantify body fat, muscle, and bone mass and total body water. In children with CP, body composition is altered due to decreased muscle and bone mass related to decreased activity levels, as well as malnutrition and neurologic impairment. Although it was once thought that children with CP had a decreased overall fat mass,[3] more recent information suggests that children with CP have similar fat mass to children without chronic health conditions.[53] An understanding of this is important, because the children may appear very thin because of low lean body mass, but actually have an appropriate fat mass.

Reliable measurements of body composition that are easy to perform in the clinical setting would provide valuable insight into a child's nutritional status. However, at this point, there is little consensus in the literature as to the best approach to measure body composition. Research has focused on direct measures of underwater weighing, deuterium-dilution technique, dual x-ray absorptiometry (DXA), and an indirect measure, namely, bioelectrical impedance (BIA). Of these methods, BIA holds promise as a technique to measure body composition that can be incorporated into clinical practice because of ease of use and its noninvasive technique.[54] BIA correlates quite well with DXA in the assessment of fat mass, as does the computing of fat mass by using the TSF and subscapular fat-fold measurements in the CP-specific equations.[50,51] At this point, the other methods are largely used on a research basis because of time constraints and lack of availability of equipment.[53]

NUTRITIONAL INTERVENTION
Enhancing Oral Nutrition

Once families and care providers decide that a concerted nutritional intervention is required for a child because of poor weight gain, depleted fat reserves, or faltering growth, a plan can be developed that focuses on improving all aspects of oral feeding, incorporates the families' priorities for feeding, and defines time frames for evaluating the efficacy of the oral nutritional rehabilitation plan (**Table 2**).

The next step is to establish specific nutrient requirements. The protein and micronutrient requirements of children with CP are similar to their age-matched peers. Special attention should be given to meeting vitamin D and calcium requirements for bone health reasons, especially for children who are not ambulant. There are, however, no standard methods for determining energy requirements for children with CP. This is in large part because of the heterogeneity of the children with CP, the high variability in

Table 2 Goals of nutrition rehabilitation	
Nutrition rehabilitation goals for children with poor nutritional status: Safe, comfortable, pleasurable intake to meet nutritional and energy requirements	
Nutrients	• Protein and micronutrients similar to requirements of age-matched peers • Meet age-appropriate calcium and vitamin D requirements • There are no clear standards for energy requirements but they are lower in children who are not ambulant than in typically growing children
Triceps skin fold	Aim for 10th–25th percentile for age
Weight	Monitor weight at 2–4-wk intervals
Weight gain velocity	Aim for 4–7 g per day in children >1 y (adjust as needed depending on degree of malnutrition)
Weight for age on cerebral palsy growth chart[10]	Aim for a weight >20th percentile which is above the "zone of concern"

motor activity, and the variations in body composition.[25] As a starting point in oral nutrition rehabilitation, care providers may want to consider increasing the caloric intake by 10% above the children's current intake. Then the anthropometric measurements can be monitored and adjustments made with the family, nutrition goals, and the time frames taken into consideration.

Food records are not useful for calculating exact intakes, because families frequently overestimate the child's intake and underestimate the amount of food lost from the child's mouth.[55] However, food records may be useful in identifying opportunities for improving the calorie and nutrient content of foods listed in the food record with nutrient-dense and high-energy food stuffs, especially fats, dairy products, sugars, and glucose polymers, commercial meal replacements, or supplements.

Oral nutritional rehabilitation involves increasing a child's caloric and nutrient intake and improving the entire feeding process. Members of the multidisciplinary team can advise families about feeding safety and efficiency[56] and about other aspects of feeding, as noted in **Box 7**.

Unfortunately, improving the nutritional status of children with significant motor impairment by oral means alone is challenging even when attention is paid to all aspects of the feeding process. Nutrition support via gastrostomy tube (GT) feeding has become widely accepted if nutrition goals cannot be met by oral means. **Box 8** describes factors to consider before GT placement.

Gastrostomy Tube Feeding

Expertise in the management of enteral feeding via GTs and the availability of appropriate devices and nutritional formulas, have contributed to the improved ability to provide nutritional rehabilitation to children with CP. However, families experience considerable decisional uncertainty regarding GT placement, because they and their children often value oral feeding despite the significant challenges that may accompany it. **Box 9** details factors that help decrease a family's decisional uncertainty about GT placement.

Although families often have considerable uncertainty about GT placement initially, they generally experience high satisfaction rates and the children generally have improved nutritional indicators and better health after GT placement (**Box 10**).

Despite the challenges with weight gain seen in children with CP who are orally fed, GT feeding can lead to an unexpectedly rapid weight gain.[60] Overnourishing children with CP puts them at a mechanical disadvantage, decreasing their already limited mobility and increasing their respiratory effort, as they have to breathe against an increased fat mass. In addition, their families experience increased strain on their backs and joints.[60,61] Frequent monitoring of the children's weight, weight gain velocity, and TSF after GT placement ensures that the child's overall growth and

---

Box 7
Other interventions for oral nutritional rehabilitation

- Positioning for optimal feeding
- Adjusting the consistency and viscosity of foods/liquids to best suit the child's skills and sensorimotor requirements
- Pacing of the feeding
- Balancing fatigue with the pleasure of eating
- The appropriate use of adaptive equipment

Box 8
Factors that warrant consideration of gastrostomy tube (GT) placement

- Prolonged meal times are limiting the child's participation in school and community activities
- Stress with the oral-feeding process is present for the child and the family
- Aspiration during feeding is interfering with pleasure of eating or is contributing to recurrent respiratory illnesses
- Ongoing poor weight gain and growth despite attempts at oral nutritional rehabilitation

---

nutritional status is improved[7] while avoiding the negative consequences of overnutrition.

Calculating calorie requirements after GT placement in children with CP can be a challenge. In general, children who require GT placement have significant motor impairments, and thus have lower energy requirements than children who are unaffected. After GT placement, some clinicians estimate caloric requirements of a child with CP to be 50% to 70%[23,61] of those a typically growing child of the same age may require. Energy requirements, as published by various national bodies[62,63] or by WHO[64] for typically growing children, can be used for these calculations. Starting with a low caloric intake, which can be increased depending on weight gain velocity and carefully monitored anthropometric measurements (see **Table 2**), has the advantage that the tube feeding may be better tolerated from the onset and that weight gain will not be excessive. Weighing the children within 2 weeks of GT placement and then monthly until the dietary requirements become clear, allows frequent fine-tuning of the nutrient intake. Dietary changes should be made by 5% to 10% increments of the total caloric intake, always ensuring the protein, vitamin D, and micronutrient intake is adequate. This can be challenging when very low caloric intakes are required. Once the appropriate nutritional goals have been achieved, monitoring of the children's nutritional status with complete anthropometric measurements should occur every 6 to 12 months.

CASE EXAMPLE

Harley was born at 26 weeks' gestation and experienced a stormy neonatal course and prolonged hospitalization. He eventually transitioned to oral feeding, but his growth and nutrition remained challenging. At 3 years of age he has CP (GMFCS 5) demonstrating spasticity and very limited mobility. Although he remains in good health and free of lower respiratory tract infections, he is falling farther behind on the conventional growth charts. His day care workers are having increasing difficulty feeding him, noting that he coughs frequently when drinking liquids, which are primarily bottle-fed. Oral food processing is minimal. His parents state that he enjoys eating the pureed foods they feed him and rarely refuses a meal, although they spend up to 6 hours a day feeding him. The food record details that he drinks 16 ounces of whole milk daily,

---

Box 9
Factors facilitating decision-making regarding GT placement for families

- Providing information without exerting pressure to make a decision
- Reassuring parents that some oral feeding can continue after GT placement
- Education about the GT simply as an adaptive device to facilitate feeding

---

Box 10
Findings after GT placement

Parents experience the following:

- High satisfaction rates with enteral feeding

- Decreased stress

- Decreased time spent feeding[57]

- Improved perception of their child's health[57,58]

Children demonstrate the following:

- Improvement in nutritional indicators

- Improved health

- Decreased hospitalization rates for pneumonia[59]

---

and eats some yogurt, infant cereal, and pureed table foods. The parents estimate that he consumes 1500 kilocalories per day, although the mealtime observation shows that the amount eaten is significantly less than reported because of loss of large quantities of food from Harley's mouth while he is eating. He is quite constipated and regurgitates once weekly, often when coughing. His only medication is vitamin D.

Harley looks very thin. He is smiling and interactive. His skin and hair are healthy, although there is an area of redness, but no skin breakdown, over the coccyx. Positive physical findings are limited to signs of his underlying disability and dental caries, in part related to the prolonged bottle-feeding and due to his inability to clear his mouth after he swallows, leaving a residue of food on his teeth. His parents are able to position him well in a specialized chair where he is fully supported for feeding. The feeding observation reveals significant oro-motor and swallowing challenges and a prolonged feeding time. Despite this, Harley and his parents clearly enjoy the feeding experience.

Harley's anthropometrics reveal a weight of 10 kg and height of 80 cm extrapolated from a knee height measurement of 20.7 cm ($20.7 \times 2.69 + 24.2$). When these are plotted on the WHO growth charts, the weight is at the 0 percentile ($z = -3.01$) and the height is at the 0 percentile ($z = -4.34$). Over time, the z-scores of his weight and height show a steady increase in distance from normal z-scores. The percentile charts have always been at or below 0 and thus provide less insight into the deviation of the basic anthropometric measurements from that of typically growing children than the z-scores. The BMI does not contribute to the assessment because it is at the 50th percentile, which is not in keeping with the clinical observation. His TSF is 5 mm, which is less than the third percentile ($z = -2$) (WHO Child Growth Standards), and his MAC of 135 mm is at the third percentile ($z = -2$) (WHO Child Growth Standards). On the CP growth charts stratified for age, degree of motor involvement, and tube feeding status, his weight-for-age plots less than the 20th percentile in the "zone of concern," where increased morbidity and mortality may result because of his nutritional status.

Harley's parents accept the information about his feeding challenges and nutrition but state at the outset that their goal is to continue oral feeding. However, together with his community therapists, day care workers, and the multidisciplinary feeding team, they participate in developing a feeding plan that addresses the following:

- Feeding safety through positioning, thickening of the fluids, pacing the liquid and solid intake, limiting the feeding time to avoid fatigue without jeopardizing intake of calories, and appropriate cup and spoon use

- Caloric and nutrient density of his foods: infant cereal, high-fat dairy products, high-fat spreads
- Managing the constipation to improve comfort
- Dental care to decrease the bacterial burden of the saliva should it be aspirated

The parents are informed about enteral feeding options, but are reticent about considering them, citing that he has been completely healthy despite the challenges.

Six weeks later, there is a bit of weight gain (2 g per day where >4 g per day would be expected for age), but the TSF is essentially unchanged, as is the weight for age (z-score now −3.03). But the parents are heartened by the small gain and wish to proceed with oral nutritional rehabilitation for 6 months. Within that time period, Harley gets an intercurrent viral illness with fever and coughing. He refuses oral intake and experiences rapid-onset dehydration and requires hospitalization. At this point, his weight is lower than it was at the start of the nutritional rehabilitation, despite the significant input of time and energy of a number of individuals. The parents become very worried about possible impact of poor nutrition on Harley's health status and the risk of dehydration because of his tenuous oral intake and consent to GT placement, which takes place when he has recovered from the intercurrent infection.

Weight gain ensues after GT feeding is initiated, even with only 500 calories per day given enterally, which is only 50% of the calories another child his age may require. Oral feeding is limited to tastes for pleasure and skill maintenance. Weekly weights during the first month after GT placement allow frequent adjustments of calorie and nutrient intake. The team decides on a maximum weight gain velocity of 10 g per day until he has achieved a TSF of the 15th percentile for age (6.25 cm) and weight of 12 kg, at which he no longer plots less than the 20th percentile on the CP growth charts (now using the ones for a boy GMFCS 5 who is tube fed).[10]

Although his parents had a difficult time deciding on GT placement, they are pleased with the outcome. They continue to feed him small amounts of pleasurable food, but use the GT for the bulk of his calories. His day care staff is pleased with the decreased coughing at meals because of the smaller intake of oral food and feel that Harley is more interested in his environment and no longer looks as fragile as he did in the past.

SUMMARY

Children with CP frequently experience challenges with nutrition and growth, which have a negative impact on their health, neurodevelopmental outcome, and survival. Intervention strategies to remediate the poor nutrition in children with CP are shaped by the following:

- Understanding of the nutritional and non-nutritional factors affecting nutrition
- Careful assessment of the nutritional status with appropriate anthropometric measures and growth charts
- Consideration of the multidimensional aspects of feeding
- Important contribution of family members in setting goals and carrying out the nutritional intervention

If nutritional rehabilitation by oral means is not successful, careful consideration must be given to providing enteral nutrition support. The decision to proceed with gastrostomy placement is frequently associated with uncertainty for families, who require considerable support to make informed decisions about the procedure. Although gastrostomy feeding is not a panacea for all nutritional problems, weight gain usually can be achieved in children with malnutrition. Although more research is required regarding nutritional rehabilitation, the hope is that early attention to the nutritional status of children with CP will translate into positive outcomes.

ACKNOWLEDGMENTS

The author thanks Dr Paul Shelton for his helpful suggestions when reviewing this article.

REFERENCES

1. Rosenbaum P, Rosenbloom L. Cerebral palsy: from diagnosis to adult life. London: MacKeith Press; 2012.
2. Rosenbaum P, Paneth M, Leviton A, et al. Definition and classification document. In: The definition and classification of cerebral palsy. Baxter P, editor. Dev Med Child Neurol Suppl 2007;109:8–14.
3. Stallings VA, Cronk CE, Zemel BS, et al. Body composition in children with spastic quadriplegic cerebral palsy. J Pediatr 1995;126:833–9.
4. Stevenson R, Hayes R, Cater L, et al. Clinical correlates of linear growth in children with cerebral palsy. Dev Med Child Neurol 1994;36:135–42.
5. Dahlseng M, Finbraten A, Juliusson R, et al. Feeding problems, growth and nutritional status in children with cerebral palsy. Acta Paediatr 2012;101:92–8. http://dx.doi.org/10.1111/j.1651-2227.2011.02412.x.
6. Kuperminc M, Stevenson R. Growth and nutrition disorders in children with cerebral palsy. Dev Disabil Res Rev 2008;14:137–46. http://dx.doi.org/10.1002/ddrr.14.
7. Andrew MJ, Sullivan PB. Growth in cerebral palsy. Nutr Clin Pract 2010;25:357–61. http://dx.doi.org/10.1177/0884533610374061.
8. Rogers B. Feeding method and health outcome of children with cerebral palsy. J Pediatr 2004;145:S28–32.
9. Samson-Fang L, Fung E, Stallings VA, et al. Relationship of nutritional status to health and societal participation in children with cerebral palsy. J Pediatr 2002;141:637–43.
10. Brooks J, Day S, Shavelle R, et al. Low weight, morbidity and mortality in children with cerebral palsy: new clinical growth charts. Pediatrics 2011;128:e299–307. http://dx.doi.org/10.1542/peds.2010-2801.
11. Samson-Fang L, Stevenson R. Linear growth velocity in children with cerebral palsy. Dev Med Child Neurol 1998;40:689–92.
12. Dahl M, Thommessen M, Rasmussen M, et al. Feeding and nutritional characteristics in children with moderate or severe cerebral palsy. Acta Paediatr 1996;85:697–701.
13. Liptak GS, O'Donnell M, Conaway M, et al. Health status of children with moderate to severe cerebral palsy. Dev Med Child Neurol 2001;43:364–70.
14. Karagiozoglu-Lampoudi T, Daskalou E, Vargiami E, et al. Identification of feeding risk factors for impaired nutrition status in paediatric patients with cerebral palsy. Acta Paediatr 2012;101:649–54.
15. Stevenson RD, Conaway M, Chumlea WC, et al. Growth and health in children with moderate-to-severe cerebral palsy. Pediatrics 2006;118:1010–8.
16. Stallings VA, Zemel BS, Davies JC, et al. Energy expenditure of children and adolescents with severe disabilities: a cerebral palsy model. Am J Clin Nutr 1996;64:627–34.
17. Andrew M, Parr J, Sullivan P. Feeding difficulties in children with CP. Arch Dis Child Educ Pract Ed 2012;97:222–9. http://dx.doi.org/10.1136/archdischild-2011-300914.

18. Sullivan RB, Lambert B, Rose M, et al. Prevalence and severity of feeding and nutritional problems in children with neurological impairment: Oxford Feeding Study. Dev Med Child Neurol 2000;42:674–80.

19. Troughton KE, Hill AE. Relation between objectively measured feeding competence and nutrition in children with cerebral palsy. Dev Med Child Neurol 2001;43:187–90.

20. Fung E, Samson-Fang L, Stallings V, et al. Feeding dysfunction is associated with poor growth and health status in children with cerebral palsy. J Am Diet Assoc 2002;102:361–73.

21. Sullivan PB, Juszczak E, Lambert BR, et al. Impact of feeding problems on nutritional intake and growth: Oxford feeding study II. Dev Med Child Neurol 2002;44: 461–7.

22. Sullivan PB. Gastrointestinal disorders in children with neurodevelopmental disabilities. Dev Disabil Res Rev 2008;14:128–36. http://dx.doi.org/10.1002/ddrr.18.

23. Walker J, Bell K, Boyd R, et al. Energy requirements in preschool-age children with CP. Am J Clin Nutr 2012;96:1309–15. http://dx.doi.org/10.3945/ajcn.112. 043430.

24. Bell KL, Samson-Fang L. Nutritional management of children with cerebral palsy. Eur J Clin Nutr 2013;67:513–6.

25. Rieken R, Goudoever J, Schierbeek H, et al. Measuring body composition and energy expenditure in children with severe neurologic impairment and intellectual disability. Am J Clin Nutr 2011;94:759–66. http://dx.doi.org/10.3945/ajcn.110. 003798.

26. Krick J, Murphy PE, Markham JF, et al. A proposed formula for calculating energy needs of children with cerebral palsy. Dev Med Child Neurol 1992;34:481–7.

27. Arrowsmith FR, Allen JK, Gaskin KG, et al. Nutritional rehabilitation increases the resting energy expenditure of malnourished children with severe cerebral palsy. Dev Med Child Neurol 2012;54:170–5. http://dx.doi.org/10.1111/j.1469-8749. 2011.04166.x.

28. Stevenson RD, Roberts CD, Vogtle L. The effects of non-nutritional factors on growth in cerebral palsy. Dev Med Child Neurol 1995;37:124–30.

29. Oeffinger D, Conaway M, Stevenson R, et al. Tibial length growth curves for ambulatory children and adolescents with cerebral palsy. Dev Med Child Neurol 2010;52:e195–201. http://dx.doi.org/10.1111/j.1469-8749.2010.03711.x.

30. Coniglio S, Stevenson R, Rogol A. Apparent growth hormone deficiency in children with cerebral palsy. Dev Med Child Neurol 1996;38:797–804.

31. Kuperminc M, Gurka M, Houlihan CM, et al. Puberty, statural growth, and growth hormone release in children with cerebral palsy. J Pediatr Rehabil Med 2009;2: 131–41. http://dx.doi.org/10.3233/PRM-2009-0072.

32. Stallings VA, Charney EG, Davies JC, et al. Nutrition-related growth failure of children with quadriplegic cerebral palsy. Dev Med Child Neurol 1993;35:126–38.

33. Rempel GR, Colwell SO, Nelson RP. Growth in children with cerebral palsy fed via gastrostomy. Pediatrics 1988;82:857–62.

34. Mehta N, Corkins M, Lyman B, et al. Defining pediatric malnutrition: a paradigm shift toward etiology-related definitions. JPEN J Parenter Enteral Nutr 2013;37: 460–81. http://dx.doi.org/10.1177/0148607113479972. Available at: http://pen. sagepub.com/content/early/2013/03/33/0148607113479972.

35. Cheong J, Hunt R, Anderson P, et al. Head growth in preterm infants: correlation with magnetic resonance imaging and neurodevelopmental outcome. Pediatrics 2008;121:e1534–40. http://dx.doi.org/10.1542/peds.2007-2671. Available at: http://pediatrics.apppublications.org/content/121/6/e1534.full.html.

36. Dabydeen L, Thomas JE, Aston TJ, et al. High-energy and -protein diet increases brain and corticospinal tract growth in term and preterm infants after perinatal brain injury. Pediatrics 2008;121:148–56. http://dx.doi.org/10.1542/peds.2007-1267. Available at: http://pediatrics.apppublications.org/content/121/1/148.full.html.

37. Campanozzi A, Capano G, Miele E, et al. Impact of malnutrition on gastrointestinal disorders and gross motor abilities in children with cerebral palsy. Brain Dev 2007;29:25–9.

38. Henderson R, Kairalla J, Abbas A, et al. Predicting low bone density in children and young adults with quadriplegic cerebral palsy. Dev Med Child Neurol 2004; 46:416–9.

39. Marchand V, Motil K, NASPGHAN Committee on Nutrition. Nutrition support for neurologically impaired children: a clinical report of the North American Society for Pediatric Gastroenterology, Hepatology, and Nutrition. J Pediatr Gastroenterol Nutr 2006;43:123–35.

40. Stevenson R, Conaway M, Barrington MK, et al. Fracture rate in children with cerebral palsy. Pediatr Rehabil 2006;9:396–403.

41. Strauss DJ, Shavelle RM, Anderson TW. Life expectancy of children with cerebral palsy. Pediatr Neurol 1998;18:143–9.

42. Strauss D, Brooks J, Rosenbloom L, et al. Life expectancy in cerebral palsy: an update. Dev Med Child Neurol 2008;50:487–93. http://dx.doi.org/10.1111/j.1469-8749.2008.03000.x.

43. Strauss D, Shavelle R, Reynolds R, et al. Survival in cerebral palsy in the last 20 years: signs of improvement? Dev Med Child Neurol 2007;49:86–92.

44. Stevenson RD. Use of segmental measure to estimate stature in children with cerebral palsy. Arch Pediatr Adolesc Med 1995;149:658–62.

45. Chumlea WC. Prediction of stature from knee height for black and white adults and children with application to mobility-impaired or handicapped persons. J Am Diet Assoc 1994;94:1385–90.

46. Stevenson RD, Conaway MR. Weight and mortality rater: "Gomez classification" for children with cerebral palsy? Pediatrics 2011;128:e436–7. http://dx.doi.org/10.1542/peds.2011-1472.

47. Samson-Fang L, Stevenson R. Identification of malnutrition in children with cerebral palsy: poor performance of weight-for-height centiles. Dev Med Child Neurol 2000;42:162–8.

48. Frisancho AT. New norms of upper limb fat and muscle areas for assessment of nutritional status. Am J Clin Nutr 1981;34:2540–5.

49. World Health Organization. Growth charts. Available at: http://www.who.int/childgrowth/standards/ac_for_age/en/. Accessed April 28, 2014.

50. Gurka M, Kuperminc M, Busby M, et al. Assessment and correction of skinfold thickness equations in estimating body fat in children with cerebral palsy. Dev Med Child Neurol 2010;52:e35–41. http://dx.doi.org/10.1111/j.1469-8749.2009.03474.x.

51. Oeffinger D, Gurka M, Kuperminc M, et al. Accuracy of skinfold and bioelectrical impedance assessment of body fat percentage in ambulatory individuals with cerebral palsy. Dev Med Child Neurol 2014;56:475–81. http://dx.doi.org/10.1111/dmcn.12342.

52. Palisano R, Rosenbaum P, Walter S, et al. Development and reliability of a system to classify gross motor function in children with cerebral palsy. Dev Med Child Neurol 1997;39:214–23.

53. Kuperminc M, Gurka M, Bennis J, et al. Anthropometric measures: poor predictors of body fat in children with moderate to severe cerebral palsy. Dev Med Child Neurol 2010;52:824–30. http://dx.doi.org/10.1111/j.1469-8749.2010.03694.x.

54. Bell KL, Boyd RN, Walker JK, et al. The use of bioelectrical impedance analysis to estimate total body water in young children with cerebral palsy. Clin Nutr 2013;32: 579–84. http://dx.doi.org/10.1016/j.clnu.2012.10.005.

55. Walker J, Bell K, Caristo F, et al. A review of energy intake measures used in young children with cerebral palsy. Dev Med Child Neurol 2011;53:569–72. http://dx.doi.org/10.1111/j.1469-8749.2011.03988.x.

56. Snider L, Majnemer A, Darsaklis V. Feeding interventions for children with cerebral palsy: a review of the evidence. Phys Occup Ther Pediatr 2011;31(1): 58–77. http://dx.doi.org/10.3109/01942638.2010.523397. Available at: http://informahealthcare.com/potp.

57. Sullivan PB, Juszczak E, Bachlet A, et al. Gastrostomy tube feeding in children with cerebral palsy: a prospective longitudinal study. Dev Med Child Neurol 2005;47:77–85.

58. Mahant S, Friedman JN, Connolly B, et al. Tube feeding and quality of life in children with severe neurological impairment. Arch Dis Child 2009;94:668–73. http://dx.doi.org/10.1136/adc.2008.149542.

59. Sullivan PB, Morrice JS, Vernon-Roberts A, et al. Does gastrostomy tube feeding in children with cerebral palsy increase the risk of respiratory morbidity? Arch Dis Child 2006;91:478–82.

60. Sullivan PB, Alder N, Bachlet AM, et al. Gastrostomy feeding in cerebral palsy: too much of a good thing? Dev Med Child Neurol 2006;48:877–82.

61. Vernon-Roberts A, Wells J, Grant H, et al. Gastrostomy feeding in cerebral palsy: enough and no more. Dev Med Child Neurol 2010;52:1099–105. http://dx.doi.org/10.1111/j.1469-8749.2010.03789.x.

62. Office of Disease Prevention and Health Promotion. Dietary guidelines for Americans. Available at: www.health.gov/dietaryguidelines/. Accessed May 27, 2014.

63. Health Canada: estimated caloric requirements. Available at: http://www.hc-sc.gc.ca/fn-an/food-guide-aliment/basics-base/1_1_1-eng.php. Accessed May 27, 2014.

64. World Health Organization. Human energy and protein requirements: report of a Joint FAO/WHO/UNU Expert Consultation. Available at: http://www.who.int/nutrition/publications/nutrientrequirements/9251052123/en/. Accessed May 27, 2014.

Pathophysiology of Muscle Contractures in Cerebral Palsy

Margie A. Mathewson, PhD[a], Richard L. Lieber, PhD[b,c],*

KEYWORDS

- Cerebral palsy • Skeletal muscle • Extracellular matrix • Sarcomere • Fiber
- Gene expression • Pathophysiology

KEY POINTS

- Muscle from patients with cerebral palsy shows functional deficits such as decreased force production and range of motion.
- Muscle is altered at a structural level, with decreased muscle body size, smaller-diameter fibers, and highly stretched sarcomeres (the force-producing unit of muscle).
- Muscle from patients with cerebral palsy has altered extracellular matrix and connective tissue.
- Decreased muscle stem cell numbers and altered gene expression have been reported in cerebral palsy.

INTRODUCTION

Nature of the Problem

Cerebral palsy (CP) is a motor disorder caused by a nonprogressive injury to the developing brain.[1] The injury occurs perinatally and, though causes are rarely known,[2,3] CP is common in infants born preterm with small birth weights.[4] CP occurs in 2 to 3 of every 1000 live births[5] and has heterogeneous symptoms, anatomic involvement, and functional impairment, including lifelong changes in motor function.[1,2] These

Disclosure: Research reported in this publication was supported by the National Institute of Arthritis and Musculoskeletal and Skin Diseases of the National Institutes of Health under Award numbers AR057393 and R24HD050837. The content is solely the responsibility of the authors and does not necessarily represent the official views of the National Institutes of Health.
[a] Department of Bioengineering, University of California San Diego, 9500 Gilman Drive, La Jolla, CA 92093-0412, USA; [b] Department of Orthopaedic Surgery, University of California San Diego, 9500 Gilman Drive, La Jolla, CA 92093-0863, USA; [c] Department of Veteran's Affairs, 3350 La Jolla Village Dr., San Diego, CA, 92161, USA
* Corresponding author. Department of Orthopaedic Surgery, University of California, San Diego, 9500 Gilman Drive, La Jolla, CA, 92093-0863.
E-mail addresses: rlieber@ric.org; rlieber@ucsd.edu

Phys Med Rehabil Clin N Am 26 (2015) 57–67
http://dx.doi.org/10.1016/j.pmr.2014.09.005
1047-9651/15/$ – see front matter Published by Elsevier Inc.

alterations stem from both changes in the neural drive to muscles[6] and changes to muscles themselves.

Symptoms

Spastic CP, which involves injury to the pyramidal system, is the most common form of CP, making up nearly 75% of all cases.[3] Spasticity has been defined as a "velocity dependent resistance to stretch."[7] Limb involvement varies, with patients showing symptoms in either all 4 limbs (tetraplegia or quadriplegia), primarily on one side of the body including one upper and lower extremity (hemiplegia), or primarily in the lower extremities (diplegia).[8] Patients' functional mobility can be classified using several rating scales, including the Gross Motor Function Classification System (GMFCS), which rates patient mobility on a scale of 1 to 5 from high to low function, respectively.[1,3] Although the injury associated with CP initially occurs in the developing brain, symptoms are commonly treated at the muscle level. Because the population affected with CP is large and heterogeneous, a better understanding, especially among clinicians and therapists, of muscular adaptations in CP may lead to improvements in treatment or even development of completely novel therapeutic strategies.

To understand the adaptations that occur in muscle from CP patients, it is important to review the function of typically developing muscle.

HEALTHY SKELETAL MUSCLE STRUCTURE AND FUNCTION
Muscle Structure

The fundamental unit of muscle force production is the sarcomere. Sarcomeres produce force by the interaction between 2 proteins, actin and myosin. Force production is affected by both muscle velocity and the amount of overlap between these 2 proteins, or sarcomere length. The sarcomere length-tension relationship has been characterized in the length-tension curve.[9] Sarcomeres are joined end to end (in series) to form myofibrils. Bundles of myofibrils form myofibers, or multinucleated muscle cells. These muscle fibers are joined into muscle fiber bundles, or fascicles (**Fig. 1**).

At each increasing size scale, extracellular matrix (ECM), the surrounding connective tissue, encapsulates muscle structures. Endomysium surrounds individual myofibers,[10] perimysium surrounds muscle fascicles,[11] and epimysium surrounds the whole muscle (see **Fig. 1**).[12,13] The composition and arrangement of these structures is important to muscle function, and can vary in muscle disorders.

The extensive growth and regeneration capacity seen in muscle is due to its intrinsic stem cell population. Most of these stem cells are called satellite cells[14] and are found below the basal lamina of myofibers; they are normally quiescent except when activated during times of muscle disease or injury.[15] Satellite cell number and viability, rather than being constant throughout life, decreases with age or diseases that are characterized by extensive regeneration.[16] Conditions such as muscular dystrophy, which require constant regeneration of muscle fibers, are believed to eventually lead to exhaustion of the satellite cell population[17] and the concomitant loss in a muscle's ability to adapt to the new functional demand.

Plasticity

Muscle has strong regenerative capacity, and can respond and change based on functional demands; for example, muscle fibers atrophy (leading to a decrease in muscle fiber size) when subject to decreased use, aging, and some diseases. Serial sarcomere number can also change in response to growth[18] as well as limb immobilization with the muscle in a shortened or lengthened position. This serial change in sarcomere

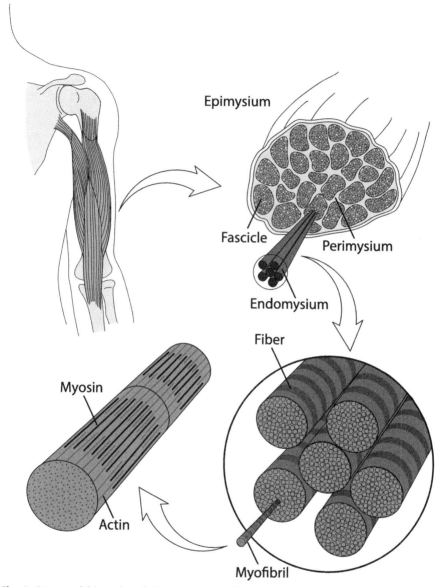

Fig. 1. Structural hierarchy of skeletal muscle. Skeletal muscle is composed of bundles of muscle fibers called fascicles. Individual fibers in these fascicles consist of myofibrils, which are composed of the contractile proteins actin and myosin. Connective tissue, which surrounds the muscle at many levels, is organized into epimysium, surrounding the whole muscle; perimysium, surrounding fascicles; and endomysium, surrounding muscle fibers. (*Modified from* Lieber RL. Skeletal muscle structure and function. Philadelphia: Lippincott Williams and Wilkins, 2010; with permission.)

number resulting from chronic change in muscle length was shown in several classic studies in both mouse[19] and cat.[20] These muscles, immobilized in a shortened position, rapidly adjust their sarcomere number to restore sarcomere length to previous values. A similar response was reported in a human case study of distraction osteogenesis in which a leg-length discrepancy was corrected as a patient's bone was gradually lengthened over time.[21] Sarcomere lengths were measured and sarcomere number calculated over the course of the treatment. As stretching of the bone and muscle occurred, sarcomere number rapidly increased and sarcomere length nearly returned to the pretreatment value.[21] Serial sarcomere number from patients with CP appears to be altered in comparison with typically developing muscles, however, suggesting that the plasticity seen in typically developing muscles may not be present to the same extent in CP.

MUSCLE PATHOLOGY OF CEREBRAL PALSY
Force Production and Muscle Function

Alterations in gait, balance, and force production have been reported for patients with CP.[22–26] For example, knee extensor force decreases with CP, which can significantly inhibit mobility.[22] Voluntary force production in general is decreased, as shown by many investigators.[27–29] There is also evidence that greater cocontraction, or simultaneous activation of a muscle and its antagonist, occurs in CP.[30] Compounding the problem of decreased force production, ankle stiffness was also shown to be 51% higher in CP, indicating increased resistance to passive ankle flexion.[31]

Muscle Architecture

Muscles in spastic CP often develop contractures, whereby joint range of motion is limited and muscles appear functionally "short."[32] Many researchers have measured changes in muscle properties such as muscle belly size, muscle length, fascicle length, and sarcomere length, all of which may help to explain this observation. Ultrasonography is probably the most common tool used to describe basic muscle structural changes, such as fiber length and tissue thickness (**Fig. 2**).[33] Previous architecture studies focused primarily on the gastrocnemius muscle, an ankle plantarflexor and knee flexor that is commonly implicated in ankle equinus contractures[34] and also plays a role in knee flexion contractures. Ultrasonographic measurements show that gastrocnemius muscle volume is smaller in patients with CP. When affected and unaffected limbs were compared in hemiplegic patients, muscle volume was

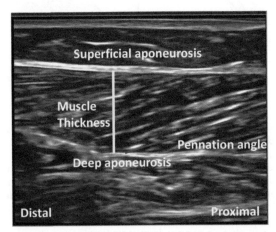

Fig. 2. Typical ultrasonography image of a human soleus muscle. Muscle appears dark and the connective tissue light on the sonogram. Superficial and deep aponeuroses surround the muscle on either side. The red line indicates the path of a muscle fascicle and the yellow line represents the thickness of the muscle belly.

decreased by 28% in the affected gastrocnemius and by nearly 50% more than muscles of typically developing children.[35] Muscle belly lengths have also been shown to decrease in CP. One 3-dimensional ultrasonography study of the medial gastrocnemius showed decreased muscle belly lengths, but no change in fascicle length when normalized to tibia length.[35] Based on the description of muscle structure presented herein, it is clear that ultrasonography alone cannot make functional predictions based on gross tissue dimensions because the composite sarcomeres cannot be detected using this modality.

In contrast to what might be expected for contractures, which are often considered permanently contracted or shortened muscles, previous fascicle length measurements in patients with CP have been inconclusive. Whereas some studies report shorter muscle fascicles in CP,[34,36] others report no difference between typically developing and CP fascicle lengths.[35,37] In contrast to the variety of results reported for fascicle length, sarcomere length, the best predictor of active muscle force, has been consistently shown to be longer in CP patients (**Fig. 3**). Whereas one study questioned the functional significance of sarcomere lengthening based on force measurements across the joint range of motion,[38] previous direct studies of sarcomere length show long sarcomeres in CP in both upper[39] and lower extremity flexors.[40] It therefore appears that regulation of sarcomere length does not occur similarly in patients with typical development and those with CP, as CP sarcomeres do not maintain a relatively constant length as in normal development.

TISSUE PROPERTIES
Mechanical Properties

While CP contractures are often thought to be stiff because of muscle overactivation, there are also critical contributions to stiffness that simply result from increased

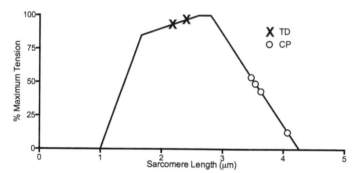

Fig. 3. Schematic length-tension curve of skeletal muscle. When sarcomere length data for cerebral palsy (CP; O symbols) and typically developing (TD; X symbols) muscles are plotted on this curve, sarcomeres clearly act in a fundamentally different region of the curve for CP in comparison with TD subjects. For example, if TD sarcomeres are stretched, maximal force production will increase, whereas the opposite will happen for CP sarcomeres. Muscles represented include gracilis, semitendinosus, soleus, and flexor carpi ulnaris. (*Data from* Mathewson MA, Ward SR, Chambers HG, et al. High resolution muscle measurements provide insights into equinus contractures in patients with cerebral palsy. J Orthop Res 2014 Sep 19. doi: 10.1002/jor.22728. [Epub ahead of print]; Lieber RL, Friden J. Spasticity causes a fundamental rearrangement of muscle-joint interaction. Muscle Nerve 2002;25(2):265–70; and Smith LR, Lee KS, Ward SR, et al. Hamstring contractures in children with spastic cerebral palsy result from a stiffer extracellular matrix and increased in vivo sarcomere length. J Physiol 2011;589(10):2625–39.)

intrinsic passive stiffness of the tissue. A recent study explored the passive mechanical properties of 2 lower extremity muscles, the semitendinosus and gracilis.[40] Fibers, whose passive mechanical properties are thought to depend mainly on the giant structural protein titin, showed similar stiffness in typically developing and CP tissue of both muscles. Titin mass was no different between the 2 groups, as would be expected from the similar fiber stiffness. Gracilis bundles were much stiffer than either typically developing bundles or bundles from the CP semitendinosus. CP semitendinosus bundles were also stiffer than their typically developing controls (**Fig. 4**). This difference in stiffness was likely due to the contributions of the ECM at the bundle level. The change in bundle stiffness between typically developing and CP tissue suggests that collagen content has increased or that there is some type of abnormal organization in the muscle ECM. Although increased collagen was observed in these muscles,[40] there are currently no tools available to quantify muscle extracellular structures accurately. Of interest, earlier studies in the upper extremity yielded very different results, reporting stiffer fibers[41] but more compliant bundles in patients with CP,[42] even though the ECM in CP muscle bundles tested in this study occupied more space than the ECM of typically developing controls.[42] The differences in stiffness among muscles, potentially resulting from differences in ECM quality and arrangement, highlight the importance of studying muscles individually rather than making generalizations, especially in the case of highly heterogeneous disorders such as CP. In addition, it is important to develop new tools that can allow accurate measurement of muscle properties that have the greatest clinical relevance.

Histology

The histologic profile of muscle from patients with CP varies (**Fig. 5A**). Although the shape of individual muscle fibers may not change as drastically as it does in some

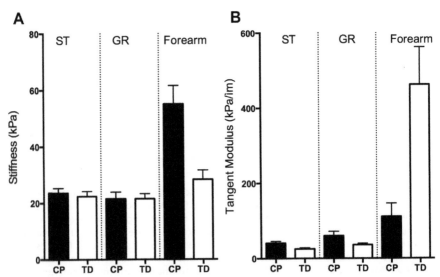

Fig. 4. Comparison between fiber and bundle stiffness in children with cerebral palsy (CP) and typically developing (TD) children. Note that axes are not the same for A and B. (*A*) Although fibers between CP and TD individuals are similar in stiffness in the gracilis (GR) and semitendinosus (ST), they are stiffer in the forearm muscles of individuals with CP. (*B*) Bundles of muscle fibers and their surrounding extracellular matrix were stiffer in CP in the GR and ST, but less stiff in the forearm. (*Data from* Refs.[40–42])

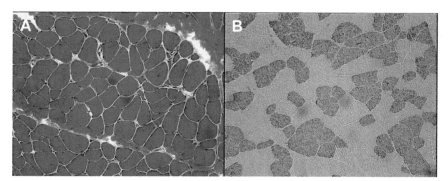

Fig. 5. Light micrographs of muscle from a patient with CP. (*A*) Hematoxylin and eosin permits evaluation of basic muscle tissue morphology (original magnification × 40). (*B*) Adenosine triphosphatase histochemical staining permits determination of muscle fiber type (original magnification × 40).

other muscular disorders, most studies report a decrease in fiber size[43,44] and an increase in variability of fiber size.[43,45] Moderate rounding of muscle fibers has also been reported.[44,45] In one study, capillary density was 30% lower in patients with CP.[46] Lipid content has been shown to increase in some cases.[43,44] Collagen content also appears to be increased,[40,45] and this has been correlated with increased stiffness of muscle fiber bundle.[40] Some investigators have even reported a significant correlation between collagen increases and patient function, using the Modified Ashworth Scale and patient balance measurements.[45]

Myosin heavy chain, the major muscle contractile protein that determines fiber type, also changes in patients with CP, although the direction of these changes varies among muscles studied and techniques used (see **Fig. 5B**). One study, using nicotinamide adenine dinucleotide (NADH) and adenosine triphosphatase (ATPase) staining, which indirectly reflect muscle oxidative capacity and contractile speed, respectively, reported increased fiber-size variability in patients with CP, and also found that patients with CP were more likely to have a strong predominance of one fiber type over the other (either type 1 or type 2). These differences were often greater than 40%, whereas typically developing patients showed no predominance.[43] Another study using similar histochemical techniques in gastrocnemius biopsies reported increases in percentage of type 1 fiber and decreases in percentage of type 2 fiber, especially histochemically defined 2B fibers.[47] In the adductor longus and triceps surea muscles, increased percentage of type 1 fiber was also reported with ATPase staining.[44] A study of hamstring muscle in which myosin isoforms were electrophoretically separated demonstrated a 30% increase in type 1 myosin heavy chain in patients with CP. However, when monoclonal antibodies were used to label different myosin heavy chain isoforms in the biceps brachii, a dramatic increase in percentage of type 2 fiber was reported, with type 2X myosin heavy chain fibers making up 30% of CP muscle compared with 4% of typically developing muscle.[46] Clearly variation exists among muscles, and further studies are needed to understand the impact of CP on predominance of muscle fiber type. From a physiologic perspective, however, percentage of fiber type is not likely to cause dramatic functional impairment, but rather reflects an altered use pattern of the muscle.

Gene Expression

Another technique used to understand muscle at the cellular level is gene expression analysis. Using microarrays, it is possible to compare thousands of genes simultaneously. Two recent studies quantified muscle genome-wide expression. The first, which compared muscles of the forearm, found distinct transcriptional differences between patients with and without CP.[48] Alterations were seen in multiple pathways, with important differences in ECM-related genes, a myosin heavy chain fiber–type shift toward faster myosin, a decrease in oxidative metabolism, and altered genes that allow excitation-contraction coupling.[48] The second study, which measured gene expression in hamstrings, found similar results, including a dramatic increase in ECM production–related gene expression (which matched the collagen

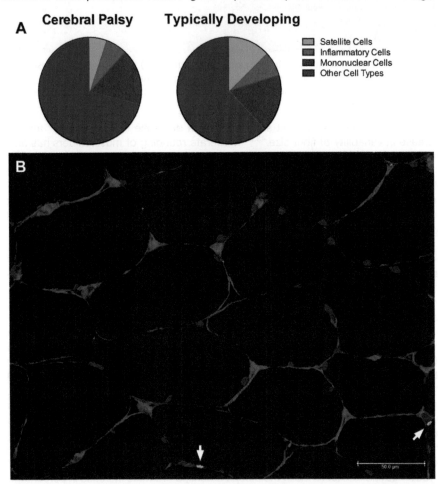

Fig. 6. Fluorescence-activated cell sorting of several muscle mononuclear populations. (*A*) Whereas the percentage of other cell types such as mononuclear cells and inflammatory cells are unchanged in patients with CP, the fraction of satellite cells in CP muscle is half of what is found in TD muscle. (*B*) Immunohistochemical image of a satellite cell is shown in its native environment. Satellite cells are identified by looking for Pax7-positive staining (*light green*) on top of a cell nucleus (4′,6-diamidino-2-phenylindole [DAPI] positive; *blue*) that is located under the basal lamina (laminin staining; *red*). Satellite cells are indicated with white arrows. ([*A*] *Data from* Smith LR, Chambers HG, Lieber RL. Reduced satellite cell population may lead to contractures in children with cerebral palsy. Dev Med Child Neurol 2013;55(3):264–70; and [*B*] *Courtesy of* the National Skeletal Muscle Research Center, San Diego, CA. Available at: http://muscle.ucsd.edu/nsmrc/home.shtml; with permission.)

content measured from the same samples) and decreased oxidative metabolism gene expression.[49] These results agree with physiologic observations in patients with CP. These transcriptional data appear to reveal "confusion" in muscle cells that exist in the CP environment.

Stem Cells

In a novel approach to understanding CP muscle, a recent publication highlighted the possible importance of certain muscle stem cells, called satellite cells, in patients with CP (**Fig. 6**). In one study, flow cytometry, a method used to count and isolate tagged cells of different types, was used to count cells in human biopsies.[50] Although there was no change in either hematopoietic or endothelial cell numbers between groups, patients with CP had fewer than half as many satellite cells when compared with typically developing control subjects (see **Fig. 6**A). This observation reveals decreased intrinsic satellite cell number or satellite cell depletion in CP, and may indicate that this change contributes to abnormal sarcomere length, changes in material properties, and contracture formation. The question as to the cellular mechanism that could explain these changes remains unanswered. However, there is the exciting possibility that should this mechanism be determined, a new therapeutic approach to curing skeletal muscle contractures might be developed.

SUMMARY

Although CP is caused by a brain injury, critical symptoms manifest in the muscle. Contractures and spasticity seen clinically correspond to changes in muscle sarcomere length, fiber type, ECM concentration, fiber and fiber bundle stiffness, and even stem cell numbers. Better understanding of muscular changes and development of new treatments that focus on these aspects might lead to new avenues for improving function in patients with CP.

REFERENCES

1. Rosenbaum P, Paneth N, Leviton A, et al. A report: the definition and classification of cerebral palsy April 2006. Dev Med Child Neurol 2007;49:8–14.
2. Bax M, Goldstein M, Rosenbaum P, et al. Proposed definition and classification of cerebral palsy. Dev Med Child Neurol 2005;47:571–6.
3. Sankar C, Mundkur N. Cerebral palsy—definition, classification, etiology and early diagnosis. Indian J Pediatr 2005;72(10):865–8.
4. Johnson A. Prevalence and characteristics of children with cerebral palsy in Europe. Dev Med Child Neurol 2002;44(09):633–40.
5. Arneson CL, Durkin MS, Benedict RE, et al. Prevalence of cerebral palsy: autism and developmental disabilities monitoring network, three sites, United States, 2004. Disabil Health J 2009;2(1):45–8.
6. Rose J, McGill KC. Neuromuscular activation and motor-unit firing characteristics in cerebral palsy. Dev Med Child Neurol 2005;47(5):329–36.
7. Tilton AH. Approach to the rehabilitation of spasticity and neuromuscular disorders in children. Neurol Clin 2003;21(4):853–81.
8. Gorter JW, Rosenbaum PL, Hanna SE, et al. Limb distribution, motor impairment, and functional classification of cerebral palsy. Dev Med Child Neurol 2004;46(7):461–7.
9. Blix M. Die lange und die spannung des muskels. Skand Arch Physiol 1894;5: 149–206.
10. Trotter JA, Purslow PP. Functional morphology of the endomysium in series fibered muscles. J Morphol 1992;212(2):109–22.

11. Rowe RW. Morphology of perimysial and endomysial connective tissue in skeletal muscle. Tissue Cell 1981;13(4):681–90.
12. Järvinen TA, Jozsa, L, Kannus, P, et al. Organization and distribution of intramuscular connective tissue in normal and immobilized skeletal muscles. J Muscle Res Cell Motil 2002;23(3):245–54.
13. Gao Y, Waas AM, Faulkner JA, et al. Micromechanical modeling of the epimysium of the skeletal muscles. J Biomech 2008;41(1):1–10.
14. Mauro A. Satellite cells of skeletal muscle fibers. J Biophys Biochem Cytol 1961; 9(2):493–5.
15. Schultz E, Gibson MC, Champion T. Satellite cells are mitotically quiescent in mature mouse muscle: an EM and radioautographic study. J Exp Zool 1978;206(3):451–6.
16. Renault V, Thornell LE, Butler-Browne G, et al. Human skeletal muscle satellite cells: aging, oxidative stress and the mitotic clock. Exp Gerontol 2002; 37(10–11):1229–36.
17. Heslop L, Morgan JE, Partridge TA. Evidence for a myogenic stem cell that is exhausted in dystrophic muscle. J Cell Sci 2000;113(12):2299–308.
18. Williams PE, Goldspink G. Longitudinal growth of striated muscle fibres. J Cell Sci 1971;9(3):751–67.
19. Goldspink G. Sarcomere length during post-natal growth of mammalian muscle fibres. J Cell Sci 1968;3(4):539–48.
20. Tabary JC, Tabary C, Tardieu C, et al. Physiological and structural changes in the cat's soleus muscle due to immobilization at different lengths by plaster casts. J Physiol 1972;224(1):231–44.
21. Boakes JL, Foran, J, Ward, SR, et al. Muscle adaptation by serial sarcomere addition 1 year after femoral lengthening. Clin Orthop Relat Res 2007;456: 250–3. http://dx.doi.org/10.1097/01.blo.0000246563.58091.af.
22. Moreau NG, Falvo MJ, Damiano DL. Rapid force generation is impaired in cerebral palsy and is related to decreased muscle size and functional mobility. Gait Posture 2012;35(1):154–8.
23. Moreau NG, Teefey SA, Damiano DL. In vivo muscle architecture and size of the rectus femoris and vastus lateralis in children and adolescents with cerebral palsy. Dev Med Child Neurol 2009;51(10):800–6.
24. Wren TA, Chatwood AP, Rethlefsen SA, et al. Achilles tendon length and medial gastrocnemius architecture in children with cerebral palsy and equinus gait. J Pediatr Orthop 2010;30(5):479–84.
25. Ballaz L, Plamondon S, Lemay M. Ankle range of motion is key to gait efficiency in adolescents with cerebral palsy. Clin Biomech 2010;25(9):944–8.
26. Abel MF, Damiano DL, Pannunzio M, et al. Muscle-tendon surgery in diplegic cerebral palsy: functional and mechanical changes. J Pediatr Orthop 1999;19(3):366–75.
27. Tammik K, Matlep M, Ereline J, et al. Quadriceps femoris muscle voluntary force and relaxation capacity in children with spastic diplegic cerebral palsy. Pediatr Exerc Sci 2008;20(1):18–28.
28. Ross SA, Engsberg JR. Relationships between spasticity, strength, gait, and the GMFM-66 in persons with spastic diplegia cerebral palsy. Arch Phys Med Rehabil 2007;88(9):1114–20.
29. Barber L, Barrett R, Lichtwark G. Medial gastrocnemius muscle fascicle active torque-length and Achilles tendon properties in young adults with spastic cerebral palsy. J Biomech 2012;45(15):2526–30.
30. Damiano DL, Quinlavin JM, Owens BF, et al. Muscle force production and functional performance in spastic cerebral palsy: relationship of cocontraction. Arch Phys Med Rehabil 2000;81(7):895–900.

31. Barber L, Barrett R, Lichtwark G. Passive muscle mechanical properties of the medial gastrocnemius in young adults with spastic cerebral palsy. J Biomech 2011;44(13):2496–500.
32. Farmer SE, James M. Contractures in orthopaedic and neurological conditions: a review of causes and treatment. Disabil Rehabil 2001;23(13):549–58.
33. Legerlotz K, Smith HK, Hing WA. Variation and reliability of ultrasonographic quantification of the architecture of the medial gastrocnemius muscle in young children. Clin Physiol Funct Imaging 2010;30(3):198–205.
34. Mohagheghi AA, Khan T, Meadows TH, et al. Differences in gastrocnemius muscle architecture between the paretic and non-paretic legs in children with hemiplegic cerebral palsy. Clin Biomech 2007;22(6):718–24.
35. Malaiya R, McNee AE, Fry NR, et al. The morphology of the medial gastrocnemius in typically developing children and children with spastic hemiplegic cerebral palsy. J Electromyogr Kinesiol 2007;17(6):657–63.
36. Mohagheghi AA, Khan T, Meadows TH, et al. In vivo gastrocnemius muscle fascicle length in children with and without diplegic cerebral palsy. Dev Med Child Neurol 2008;50(1):44–50.
37. Barber LE, Hastings-Ison T, Baker R, et al. Medial gastrocnemius muscle volume and fascicle length in children aged 2 to 5 years with cerebral palsy. Dev Med Child Neurol 2011;53(6):543–8.
38. Smeulders MJ, Kreulen M, Hage JJ, et al. Overstretching of sarcomeres may not cause cerebral palsy muscle contracture. J Orthop Res 2004;22(6):1331–5.
39. Lieber RL, Fridén J. Spasticity causes a fundamental rearrangement of muscle–joint interaction. Muscle Nerve 2002;25(2):265–70.
40. Smith LR, Ponten E, Hedstrom Y, et al. Hamstring contractures in children with spastic cerebral palsy result from a stiffer extracellular matrix and increased in vivo sarcomere length. J Physiol 2011;589(10):2625–39.
41. Fridén J, Lieber RL. Spastic muscle cells are shorter and stiffer than normal cells. Muscle Nerve 2003;27(2):157–64.
42. Lieber RL, Runesson E, Einarsson F, et al. Inferior mechanical properties of spastic muscle bundles due to hypertrophic but compromised extracellular matrix material. Muscle Nerve 2003;28(4):464–71.
43. Rose J, Haskell WL, Gamble JG, et al. Muscle pathology and clinical measures of disability in children with cerebral palsy. J Orthop Res 1994;12(6):758–68.
44. Marbini A, Ferrari A, Cioni G, et al. Immunohistochemical study of muscle biopsy in children with cerebral palsy. Brain Dev 2002;24(2):63–6.
45. Booth CM, Cortina-Borja MJ, Theologis TN. Collagen accumulation in muscles of children with cerebral palsy and correlation with severity of spasticity. Dev Med Child Neurol 2001;43(5):314–20.
46. Pontén EM, Stal PS. Decreased capillarization and a shift to fast myosin heavy chain IIx in the biceps brachii muscle from young adults with spastic paresis. J Neurol Sci 2007;253(1–2):25–33.
47. Ito J, Araki A, Tanaka H, et al. Muscle histopathology in spastic cerebral palsy. Brain Dev 1996;18(4):299–303.
48. Smith L, Ponten E, Hedstrom Y, et al. Novel transcriptional profile in wrist muscles from cerebral palsy patients. BMC Med Genomics 2009;2(1):44.
49. Smith LR, Ponten E, Hedstrom Y, et al. Transcriptional abnormalities of hamstring muscle contractures in children with cerebral palsy. PLoS One 2012;7(8):e40686.
50. Smith LR, Chambers HG, Lieber RL. Reduced satellite cell population may lead to contractures in children with cerebral palsy. Dev Med Child Neurol 2013;55(3):264–70.

Pediatric Tone Management

Sathya Vadivelu, MD[a], Anne Stratton, MD[b], Wendy Pierce, MD[c],*

KEYWORDS

- Hypertonia • Spasticity • Dystonia • Baclofen • Rhizotomy • Neurotomy
- Cerebral palsy • Pediatric

KEY POINTS

- The type of hypertonicity needs to be identified to determine optimal treatment.
- Pediatric tone management involves all individuals caring for that child, including the patient, family, therapists, and the medical team.
- There are multiple nonsurgical and surgical treatments for hypertonicity.

INTRODUCTION

Tone management is one of the primary roles of a pediatric physiatrist and is a rewarding but frequently challenging task. Hypertonicity frequently inhibits normal movement patterns in children with central nervous system (CNS) lesions. At times, hypertonicity can reinforce muscle group firing and be useful for a child's function, such as stabilizing the lower limbs during stand pivot transfers. Hypertonicity can manifest as spasticity, dystonia, or rigidity, and frequently a combination is present. The manifestations of hypertonicity, underlying etiologies, and guiding treatment principles are reviewed.

Spasticity is probably the most common and easily recognizable form of hypertonicity. Spasticity is defined as increased muscle tone where resistance to externally imposed movement increases with increased speed of stretch and varies with the direction of joint movement.[1] A child may experience difficulty with smooth movements because of spasticity. The muscle stretch reflex may be inadvertently triggered

Disclosures: None.
[a] Division of Pediatric Rehabilitation Medicine, Department of Pediatrics, Rady Children's Hospital San Diego, University of California San Diego, 3020 Children's Way MC5096, San Diego, CA 92123, USA; [b] Department of Physical Medicine and Rehabilitation, University of Colorado, Denver, CO, USA; [c] Department of Physical Medicine and Rehabilitation, University of Colorado, 4125 Briargate Parkway, Box 520, Colorado Springs, CO 80920, USA
* Corresponding author.
E-mail address: wendy.pierce@childrenscolorado.org

Phys Med Rehabil Clin N Am 26 (2015) 69–78
http://dx.doi.org/10.1016/j.pmr.2014.09.008
1047-9651/15/$ – see front matter © 2015 Elsevier Inc. All rights reserved.

during activity, and the muscle "catch" may result in loss of postural stability. A commonly used scale to grade spasticity is the Modified Ashworth Scale using a range from 0 to 4, indicating no increased tone (0) to complete resistance to movement or rigidity (4).[2]

Dystonia is a more complicated form of tone. It is characterized as increased muscle tone due to abnormal involuntary co-contractions in muscle groups causing repeated abnormal posturing of the neck, torso, or limbs.[1] Dystonia is typically characterized as primary dystonia or secondary dystonia, which is typically due to an underlying cortical lesion in the thalamus or basal ganglia.[3] Functionally, dystonia or dystonic movements increase when a child attempts to perform a novel or difficult task. Usually when the child is relaxed, there is no increased tone and all limbs may be freely mobilized. When the dystonia is active, the affected body areas or limbs twist into varied postures even when the child is performing a task with the unaffected limbs. Severe dystonia with co-contractions can present at rest with joint rigidity. Dystonia is commonly measured using the Fahn-Marsden (or Burke-Fahn-Marsden) rating scale or the Barry-Albright Dystonia Scale. The Fahn-Marsden scale ranges from 0 to 4, from no dystonia, dystonia with a particular action, dystonia on many actions, to dystonia at rest. Each limb and the trunk, head, and neck are evaluated.[4] The Barry-Albright Dystonia scale also ranges from 0 to 4, but looks at the frequency of dystonia over 8 body regions.[5]

A mixture of spasticity and dystonia is frequently present in children with more severe CNS lesions and is important to consider when treating tone disorders. Spasticity, dystonia, or a combination can lead to limb rigidity, which complicates treatment options.

Many pediatric conditions lead to hypertonicity, including cerebral palsy (CP), acquired brain injury, metabolic disorders, leukodystrophies, hydrocephalus, or spinal cord injury. CP is the most common condition associated with hypertonicity.

CP "describes a group of permanent disorders of the development of movement and posture, causing activity limitation, that are attributed to nonprogressive disturbances that occurred in the developing fetal or infant brain. The motor disorders of CP are often accompanied by disturbances of sensation, perception, cognition, communication and behavior, by epilepsy, and by secondary musculoskeletal problems."[6] Tone and disorders of movement vary greatly among the CP population but most have some difficulties with limb hypertonicity.[7,8] Cerebral vascular accidents, hypoxic ischemic events, hemorrhagic events related to extreme prematurity, traumatic brain injury, neonatal toxoplasmosis, other (syphilis, varicella-zoster, parvovirus B19), rubella, cytomegalovirus (CMV), and herpes infections (TORCH) infection, or isolated metabolic derangement injuries can lead to CP, highlighting the heterogeneity of this diagnosis. Neuronal migration abnormalities, such as schizencephaly, porencephaly, and polymicrogyria, may qualify under the CP diagnosis umbrella if no other genetic syndromes are associated.

When evaluating a child with newly noted hypertonicity, brain and spinal cord imaging should be considered to evaluate reversible etiologies. The American Academy of Neurology published a practice parameter guideline for "Diagnostic assessment of the child with cerebral palsy." This guideline summary provides levels of evidence associated with workup measures for a child with suspected CP.[9]

There are many causes of hypertonicity and a multitude of treatments to manage spasticity and dystonia. Treatment approaches should be individualized based on functional goals of the child and family, level of impairment, and/or ability to care for the child. The type, locality, and severity of hypertonicity need to be considered. Treatment plans should be created in collaboration with all individuals caring for the child, including the patient, family, therapists, and medical team.

NONSURGICAL MANAGEMENT OF HYPERTONICITY

Nonsurgical management of spasticity and dystonia ranges from physical management to systemic medications and focal injections.

Physical Management of Hypertonicity

Physical management of focal and generalized hypertonicity continues to evolve over time and includes physical therapy, occupational therapy, orthoses, casting, modalities, and assistive technology. Early-intervention studies found that initiating services before 6 months of age was most effective.[10] The most effective therapy approach for managing tone and impacting function is still unclear.

Passive stretch is a focal approach to tone management that increases range of motion and reduces spasticity.[11] Spasticity is responsive to sustained stretch over several hours.[12] Orthoses and casts are often used to reduce tone by reducing tonic stretch reflexes by prolonged static stretch.[13,14] Caution should be used with certain orthoses, such as spring-assisted dorsiflexion, as they may exacerbate rapid stretch, triggering increased spasticity. Serial casting changes the number of sarcomeres and cross-bridge attachments in muscle. Serial casting also provides constant sensory input, which modulates the response of the muscle spindle and potentially decreasing spasticity.[10]

Physical and occupational therapy techniques are based on different theories of motor learning to decrease generalized spasticity.[10,15] In 2012, Franki and colleagues[15] performed a systematic review of therapy techniques for tone management. They found neurodevelopmental treatment (NDT), functional and task-oriented training, and therapeutic horse riding or hippotherapy had Level IV evidence, hinting at the causality of reduction in spasticity. Dimitrijević and colleagues[16] found a statistically significant reduction in spasticity in children with CP who participated in a twice-weekly aquatic therapy program for 12 weeks. Constraint-induced movement therapy (CIMT) may show functional benefits, but does not statistically change upper limb spasticity.[17]

Modalities and manual therapies also have been used in attempts to reduce focal hypertonia. Therapeutic heat and ultrasound reduce tone by facilitating uptake of neurotransmitters and return of calcium to the sarcoplasmic reticulum. Therapeutic cold presumably reduces clonus by acting at the cutaneous mechanoreceptor level, which impacts interneuron excitatory presynaptic potentials at the spinal cord level.[13] Cryotherapy reduces compound motor-action potentials, which reduces spasticity, but also decreases motor performance.[10] Vibration, acupuncture, and craniosacral therapy have been used, but there are few data reflecting their efficacy on reduction of hypertonicity.[10] Electrical stimulation produces a statistically significant reduction in spasticity immediately after stimulation.[18] The effect of electrical stimulation on spasticity is thought to be due to secondary relaxation as a result of the habituation of the muscle spindle to the sensory stimulus.[10]

Enteral Medications for Management of Spasticity

Benzodiazepines, such as diazepam, facilitate CNS inhibition via potentiation of gamma-aminobutyric acid (GABA) at the spinal and supraspinal levels, leading to a reduction in spasticity, hyperreflexia, and muscle spasms.[19] Benzodiazepines also have been reported to help with sleep, decrease anxiety, and aid in management of seizures.[10] Side effects include sedation, difficulty with consolidation and formation of new memory, urinary retention, liver toxicity, and dependency.[10,19] Abrupt cessation of benzodiazepines may lead to agitation, tremor, muscle fasciculation, nausea, hyperpyrexia, and seizures. It is recommended to start with nightly dosing because of their sedating effects and titrate up to dosing twice a day to 3 times a day.[19]

Baclofen binds to GABA$_B$ receptors and inhibits release of excitatory neurotransmitters and substance P, resulting in decreased spasms, clonus, and spasticity.[19] Side effects include sedation, potential exacerbation of underlying seizure disorder, hypotonia, fatigue, nausea, and vertigo. Withdrawal from baclofen may lead to rebound spasticity, hypertension, hallucinations, seizures, and hyperpyrexia.[10,19] Although baclofen has been found to be less sedating than diazepam, it is still recommended to begin with nightly dosing and titrate up to dosing twice a day to 3 times a day.[19]

Dantrolene inhibits calcium release from the sarcoplasmic reticulum during muscle contraction. The effects are reduction in clonus and muscle spasms caused by innocuous stimuli.[19] Dantrolene can be effective in athetoid CP.[10] Side effects include mild sedation, although much less than diazepam and baclofen, malaise, nausea, vomiting, dizziness, diarrhea, and paresthesias. Hepatotoxicity can occur, so transaminase monitoring must be performed and is not dose dependent.

Tizanidine is an alpha-2 adrenergic agonist that acts at the spinal and supraspinal levels, leading to hyperpolarization of motor neurons to reduce spasticity. Side effects include sedation, hypotension, dry mouth, dizziness, and hepatotoxicity, so transaminase monitoring is recommended.

Tiagabine was originally used as an anticonvulsant, but it has been shown to be beneficial in reducing painful nocturnal spasms. It should be used with caution in those with hepatic insufficiency. Its side effects include dizziness, weakness, nausea, tremor, nervousness, confusion, difficulty with concentration, and abdominal pain. It is not recommended for children younger than 12 years.

Enteral Medications for Management of Dystonia

Much like spasticity, dystonia may be focal or generalized. Although treatment approaches for focal dystonia may include medications or focal injections, generalized dystonias in childhood should begin with a trial of dopaminergic agents. A dopa-responsive dystonia can be caused by a mutation of the GTP cyclohydrolase I gene on chromosome 14q, leading to an abnormality in dopamine synthesis. Symptoms include diurnal variation in dystonia and symptoms of parkinsonism. Dopa-responsive dystonia typically responds well to carbidopa/levodopa.[20] Its side effects include dyskinesias, bradykinesia, hypotension, hallucinations, confusion, and memory impairment.[19]

Trihexyphenidyl can be effective in the management of dystonia. Its side effects include dry mouth, blurred vision, urinary retention, anhidrosis, tardive dyskinesia, glaucoma, nausea, dizziness, anxiety, and neuroleptic malignant syndrome.[19]

Baclofen also is used to treat dystonia, especially when carbidopa/levodopa and trihexyphenidyl fail to produce an adequate response. Higher doses are generally required to manage dystonia compared with spasticity.[20]

Clonazepam, in combination with anticholinergic medications, has been helpful in treatment of myoclonus-dystonia.[20]

Tetrabenazine and zolpidem have been trialed in treatment of dystonia. Tetrabenazine is an antidopaminergic drug that has been particularly helpful with tardive dystonia, but has many side effects, including transient acute dystonic reactions, insomnia, depression, and akathisia. Zolpidem, which has a high affinity for BZ1 receptors in the basal ganglia, has been effective in helping with some forms of dystonia.[20]

Treatment for Focal Hypertonicity

In addition to physical modalities to help manage focal hypertonicity, certain medications may be injected, producing a neuromuscular blockage or chemodenervation within specific muscles to reduce focal spasticity or dystonia.

Chemodenervation through axonal degeneration may be accomplished using 3% to 5% phenol or 35% to 65% ethyl alcohol. These medications require localization using nerve stimulation or ultrasound for accurate perineural localization. The use of electric stimulation, the amount of time required for localization, and caustic effects of the medication cause pain and discomfort, especially in children, so sedation is often used. Care should be taken to avoid sensory and mixed sensorimotor nerves, because destruction of sensory fibers results in painful dysesthesias and numbness. Chemodenervation using phenol or ethyl alcohol is a cost-effective means of managing spasticity for 3 to 12 months with immediate effects.[19]

Targeted injections of 5 to 10 mL of lidocaine 0.5% may provide temporary relief in focal dystonias, writer's cramp, and oromandibular dystonias. The effects may last up to 24 hours, but can be lengthened to potentially several weeks with the addition of ethanol to the injection.[20]

Neuromuscular blockade using botulinum toxin (BoNT) has been effective in managing focal spasticity, cervical dystonia, blepharospasms, oromandibular dystonia, and task-specific dystonias. The commercially available forms include onabotulinumtoxinA, abobotulinumtoxinA, incobotulinumtoxinA, and rimabotulinumtoxinB. All active forms of botulinum toxin are made of a heavy chain that binds to the presynaptic membrane. A zinc-dependent protease light chain cleaves the SNAP-25 protein in BoNT-A or the synaptobrevin-2 protein in BoNT-B, preventing acetylcholine vesicles from docking and releasing.[20] Dosing regimens for the commercially available versions of botulinum toxin are not equivalent. The effects of botulinum toxin may be seen 5 to 7 days after injection and may last 3 to 6 months. Potential side effects include transient weakness, flulike symptoms, dysphagia, respiratory difficulties, transient ptosis, blurred vision, and hypophonia, depending on the sites injected.[19,20] It has been found to have better efficacy when used in combination with other therapies.

Treatment Combinations

In a systematic review by Sakzewski and colleagues[21] of intramuscular botulinum toxin A injections with CIMT, bimanual intensive training, or NDT; no treatment was superior. BoNT-A combined with other treatment approaches provided supplementary benefit. This was further demonstrated by Hoare and colleagues[22] in 2010, who found improvements in range of motion with administration of BoNT-A injections in conjunction with occupational therapy. In 2007, Ronan and Gold[10] found that kinesio-taping in combination with other tone-modifying agents can influence hypertonicity.

SURGICAL MANAGEMENT OF HYPERTONIA

Surgical management of the hypertonia, as with other forms of management, has to be goal-based, as mentioned. The goals need to be clearly defined before determining whether surgery is a viable option. Clearly identifying the type of movement disorder, spasticity, dystonia, or athetosis, will play a role in surgical outcome. Both orthopedic and neurosurgical procedures can be therapeutic.

Orthopedic Procedures

Orthopedic surgeries primarily correct the musculoskeletal sequelae of spasticity, specifically joint contracture, subluxation, dislocation, or rotational abnormalities.

Orthopedic procedures improve passive range of motion. The improvement of active range of motion will depend on the patient's underlying strength and level of control of the underlying movement. Current evidence suggests that single-event multilevel surgery provides better quality-of-life outcomes.[23]

After any tenotomy, there is observed short-term tone reduction. There is fibrosis and decreased responsiveness of the Golgi tendon organs in rat models.[24] Tenotomy provides an interim solution and additional methods for tone management need to continue.

Neurosurgical Procedures

Cerebellar stimulation had shown some reduction in tone in approximately 80% of patients. The theory was that stimulation of these tracts would result in inhibition of activity. Spinal cord stimulation showed limited success with some dystonias but with minimal clinical effect.

Percutaneous radiofrequency rhizotomy was attempted in the lumbar spine in the spinal cord injury population. This provided only temporary results that lasted for months.

Myelotomy involved making an incision in the gray matter of the spinal cord. This disconnects the anterior horn cell from the posterior horn, thus interrupting the reflex arc. This was very effective in patients with spinal cord injury, but patients were reluctant to consent to further damaging the spinal cord. This is not an option in CP or any acquired brain due to the potential neurogenic bowel and bladder consequences.

Selective peripheral neurotomy was first introduced in the 1980s. Using this approach, the targeted nerve is dissected; electrical stimulation is then used to identify the sensory and motor nerve fascicles that result in an increased spastic response. The technique today is being performed in the sciatic, median, ulnar, musculocutaneous, and posterior tibial nerves. Patients who are ideal candidates for this procedure have primary spasticity versus dystonia.

Berard and colleagues[25] published neurotomy outcomes in 13 exclusively pediatric patients with hemiplegia. Unfortunately, 61% of patients (8/13) had recurrence of spasticity, with 4 of 13 requiring orthopedic intervention. Of the patients who required orthopedic intervention, biopsy was performed showing evidence of reinnervation.

Kwak and colleagues[26] looked at adults with finger spasticity and followed patients for up to 42 months postoperatively. They found continued effects from surgery at follow-up. Only 1 of 22 patients had dysesthesias. Buffenoir and colleagues[27] followed 15 patients who underwent tibial neurotomy for 15 months. Ninety percent of patients had clinical reduction of spasticity. Seventy-eight percent of patients had a reduction in H responses. Eighty percent had reduction of T responses. One in 15 patients had transient heel pain that was not clearly explained. Bollens and colleagues[28] randomized 16 patients for botulinum toxin injections to the soleus, tibialis posterior, and flexor hallucis longus or for selective tibial neurotomy. Findings at 6 months demonstrated a higher reduction of viscoelastic stiffness with selective tibial neurotomy, with no significant differences in gait parameters that were measured. One patient developed hypoesthesia around the surgical scar but did not develop neuropathic pain.

Intrathecal baclofen is an approved method of treatment for spasticity as well as dystonia. The pump is routinely implanted in the abdominal wall but the recommended location may change depending on the level of central obesity and other factors. The catheter is inserted into the spinal canal, typically in the lumbar spine. The tip of the catheter is then advanced superiorly depending on the areas affected by spasticity. Dosage is titrated to effect by a trained medical professional via programming of the pump, and the pump reservoir is refilled depending on rate of use of the baclofen.

There is more pediatric than adult data available for intrathecal baclofen therapy. Complication rates published between 2 institutions include mechanical complications of 15.0% to 19.3% and infection rate of 9.3%–21.8%.[29,30] Mathur and colleagues[31] described a cohort of patients between 10 and 28 years of age who reported not only reduction in spasm frequency, but also reduction in pain associated with hypertonia with an improvement in quality of life. Baker and colleagues[32] reported an overall improvement in comfort in pediatric patients 37 months after implantation. Hoving and colleagues[33] conducted a randomized controlled trial where the treatment group was implanted 1 month after the trial and the control group was implanted 6 months after the trial. Overall, the treatment group not only had reduction of spasticity, but improvement of pain and discomfort associated with spasticity.

Although spasticity is the primary indication for intrathecal baclofen therapy, it is also an effective method of treating secondary dystonia. The first case report was in 1991 by Narayan and colleagues.[34] Motta and colleagues[35] reported improvement in dystonia in 18 of 19 patients.[36] They also reported improvement in quality of upper limb movement in 10 of 11 patients with secondary dystonia due to CP.

Dorsal rhizotomy was first introduced as a treatment for spasticity in 1913. The selective process to identify the sensory roots was introduced in the 1970s. The ideal selective dorsal rhizotomy (SDR) candidate is 3 to 6 years old with near-normal cognitive function and spastic diplegia. If the patient is ambulatory, he or she must have sufficient underlying strength so as to remain ambulatory postoperatively. Patients with primarily dystonia and athetosis are not good candidates for this procedure. Complications include transient cerebral spinal fluid leakage, dysesthesias, transient urinary retention, back pain, sensory changes, and neurogenic bowel and bladder.[37]

Long-term outcomes for SDR were recently published by Dudley and colleagues.[38] Reduction in tone was maintained up to 15 years from the time of surgery. Nordmark and colleagues[39] followed patients for 5 years with gross motor functional classification system (GMFCS) scores ranging from I to V. There were some improvements in the gross motor function measure (GMFM)-66 in those with GMFCS III to V at 18 months to 5 years. Chan and colleagues[40] looked at 20 children in Hong Kong with GMFCS levels I to III. There was an average increase of 3.8 points in the GMFM and overall improvement in the Pediatric Evaluation of Disability Inventory following SDR.

Deep brain stimulation (DBS) is a surgical treatment specifically for dystonia. It stimulates areas around the subthalamic nucleus that results in a cascade of events that modulates the basal ganglia and thalamocortical network. It is a very effective treatment for primary dystonia, Parkinson disease, and essential tremor. There are limited results in treating secondary dystonia.[41] Complications of surgery include intracerebral and intraventricular hemorrhage, ischemic infarction, hardware discomfort, loss of effect, infection, lead malposition, and component fracture and malfunction.[42]

Fitzgerald and colleagues[43] reported on a series of 60 children and adults with generalized dystonia with no improvement in secondary dystonia. Olaya and colleagues[44] published a case series of 9 children with secondary dystonia who underwent DBS implantation in the globus pallidus, demonstrating a reduction in the Barry-Albright Dystonia Scale and the Burke-Fahn-Marsden Dystonia Rating Scale.

Gimeno and colleagues[45] looked specifically at 30 children with dystonia who underwent DBS implantation. Although they reported no significant improvement in dystonia scales, there was improvement in quality-of-life measures.

In conclusion, the patient population requiring tone management is quite diverse. Patient and family goals, care-team goals, type(s) of tone being addressed, and risks and benefits should all be carefully considered when making recommendations for management. There are many options available for tone management that frequently work in combination.

REFERENCES

1. Sanger TD, Delgado MR, Gaebler-Spira D, et al. Classification and definition of disorders causing hypertonia in childhood. Pediatrics 2003;111(1):e89–97.
2. Bohannon R, Smith M. Interrater reliability of a modified Ashworth scale of muscle spasticity. Phys Ther 1987;67(2):206.
3. Berardelli A, Rothwell JC, Hallett M, et al. The pathophysiology of primary dystonia. Brain 1998;121:1195–212.
4. Burke RE, Fahn S, Marsden CD, et al. Validity and reliability of a rating scale for the primary torsion dystonias. Neurology 1985;35:73–7.
5. Albright MJ, VanSwearigen JM, Albright AL. Reliability and responsiveness of the Barry-Albright dystonia scale. Dev Med Child Neurol 1999;6:404–11.
6. Rosenbaum P, Paneth N, Leviton A, et al. A report: the definition and classification of cerebral palsy April 2006. Dev Med Child Neurol 2007;49:8–14.
7. Paneth N, Hong T, Korzeniewski S. The descriptive epidemiology of cerebral palsy. Clin Perinatol 2006;33(2):251–67.
8. Surveillance of Cerebral Palsy in Europe (SCPE). Prevalence and characteristics of children with cerebral palsy in Europe. Dev Med Child Neurol 2002;44:633–40.
9. Ashwal S, Russman BS, Blasco PA, et al, Practice Committee of the Child Neurology Society. Practice parameter: diagnostic assessment of the child with cerebral palsy: report of the Quality Standards Subcommittee of the American Academy of Neurology and the Practice Committee of the Child Neurology Society. Neurology 2004;62(6):851–63.
10. Ronan S, Gold JT. Nonoperative management of spasticity in children. Childs Nerv Syst 2007;23:943–56.
11. Wusthoff CJ, Shellhaas RA, Licht DJ. Management of common neurologic symptoms in pediatric palliative care: seizures, agitation, and spasticity. Pediatr Clin North Am 2007;54(5):709–33, xi.
12. Pin T, Dyke P, Chan M. The effectiveness of passive stretching in children with cerebral palsy. Dev Med Child Neurol 2006;48(10):855–62.
13. Parziale JR, Akelman E, Herz DA. Spasticity: pathophysiology and management. Orthopedics 1993;16(7):803–11.
14. Tardieu C, Lespargot A. For how long must the soleus muscle be stretched each day to prevent contracture? Dev Med Child Neurol 1988;30(1):3–10.
15. Franki I, Desloovere K, De Cat J, et al. The evidence-base for conceptual approaches and additional therapies targeting lower limb function in children with cerebral palsy: a systematic review using the ICF as a framework. J Rehabil Med 2012;44(5):396–405.
16. Dimitrijević L, Bjelaković B, Lazović M, et al. Aquatic exercise in the treatment of children with cerebral palsy. Srp Arh Celok Lek 2012;140(11–12):746–50.
17. Anttila H, Autti-Rämö I, Suoranta J, et al. Effectiveness of physical therapy interventions for children with cerebral palsy: a systematic review. BMC Pediatr 2008; 8:14.
18. Suh HR, Han HC, Cho HY. Immediate therapeutic effect of interferential current therapy on spasticity, balance, and gait function in chronic stroke patients: a randomized control trial. Clin Rehabil 2014;28:885–91.
19. Deon LL, Gaebler-Spira D. Assessment and treatment of movement disorders in children with cerebral palsy. Orthop Clin North Am 2010;41(4):507–17.

20. Jankovic J. Medical treatment of dystonia. Mov Disord 2013;28(7):1001–12.
21. Sakzewski L, Ziviani J, Boyd R. Systematic review and meta-analysis of thera-peutic management of upper-limb dysfunction in children with congenital hemi-plegia. Pediatrics 2009;123:e1111–22.
22. Hoare BJ, Wallen MA, Imms C, et al. Botulinum toxin A as an adjunct to treat-ment in the management of the upper limb in children with spastic cerebral palsy (UPDATE). Cochrane Database Syst Rev 2010;(1):CD003469.
23. Himpens E, Franki I, Geerts D, et al. Quality of life in youngsters with cerebral palsy after single-event multilevel surgery. Eur J Paediatr Neurol 2013;17(4): 401–6.
24. Jamali AA, Afshar P, Abrams RA, et al. Skeletal muscle response to tenotomy. Muscle Nerve 2000;23:851–62.
25. Berard C, Sindou M, Berard J, et al. Selective neurotomy of the tibial nerve in the spastic hemiplegic child: an explanation of recurrence. J Pediatr Orthop B 1998; 7(1):66–70.
26. Kwak KW, Kim MS, Chang CH, et al. Surgical results of selective median neuro-tomy for wrist and finger spasticity. J Korean Neurosurg Soc 2011;50:95–8.
27. Buffenoir K, Decq P, Hamel O, et al. Long-term neuromechanical results of selec-tive tibial neurotomy in patients with spastic equinus foot. Acta Neurochir 2013; 155:1731–43.
28. Bollens B, Gustin T, Stoquart G, et al. A randomized control trial of selective neurotomy versus botulinum toxin for spastic equinovarus foot after stroke. Neu-rorehabil Neural Repair 2014;27(8):695–703.
29. Motta F, Antonello CE. Analysis of complications in 430 consecutive pediatric pa-tients treated with intrathecal baclofen therapy: 14-year experience. J Neurosurg Pediatr 2014;13(3):301–6.
30. Ghosh D, Mainali G, Khera J, et al. Complications of intrathecal baclofen pumps in children: experience from a tertiary care center. Pediatr Neurosurg 2013;49: 138–44.
31. Mathur SN, Chu SK, McCormick Z, et al. Long-term intrathecal baclofen: out-comes after more than 10 years of treatment. PM R 2014;6:506–13.e1.
32. Baker KW, Tann B, Mutlu A, et al. Improvements in children with cerebral palsy following intrathecal baclofen: use of the Rehabilitation Institute of Chicago care and comfort caregiver questionnaire (RIC CareQ). J Child Neurol 2013; 29(3):312–7.
33. Hoving MA, van Raak EP, Spincemaille GH, et al, Dutch Study Group on Child Spasticity. Efficacy of intrathecal baclofen therapy in children with intractable spastic cerebral palsy: a randomised controlled trial. Eur J Paediatr Neurol 2009;13(3):240–6.
34. Narayan RK, Loubser PG, Jankovic J, et al. Intrathecal baclofen for intractable axial dystonia. Neurology 1991;41(7):1141–2.
35. Motta F, Antonello CE, Stignani C. Upper limb function after intrathecal baclofen therapy in children with secondary dystonia. J Pediatr Orthop 2009;29:817–21.
36. Motta F, Stignani C, Antonello CE. Effect of intrathecal baclofen on dystonia in children with cerebral palsy and the use of functional scales. J Pediatr Orthop 2008;28:213–7.
37. Steinbok P, Schraq C. Complications after selective posterior rhizotomy for spas-ticity in children with cerebral palsy. Pediatr Neurosurg 1998;28(6):300–13.
38. Dudley RW, Parolin M, Gagnon B, et al. Long-term functional benefits of selective dorsal rhizotomy for spastic cerebral palsy. J Neurosurg Pediatr 2013;12(2): 142–50.

39. Nordmark E, Josenby AL, Lagergren J, et al. Long-term outcomes five years after selective dorsal rhizotomy. BMC Pediatr 2008;14(8):54. http://dx.doi.org/10.1186/1471-2431-8-54.

40. Chan SH, Yam KY, Yiu-Lau BP, et al. Selective dorsal rhizotomy in Hong Kong: multidimensional outcome measures. Pediatr Neurol 2008;39:22–32.

41. Miocinovic S, Somayajula S, Chitnis S, et al. History, applications, and mechanisms of deep brain stimulation. JAMA Neurol 2013;70(2):163–71.

42. Fenoy AJ, Simpson RK Jr. Risks of common complications in deep brain stimulation surgery: management and avoidance. J Neurosurg 2014;120(1):132–9.

43. Fitzgerald JJ, Rosendal F, de Pennington N, et al. Long-term outcome of deep brain stimulation in generalized dystonia: a series of 60 cases. J Neurol Neurosurg Psychiatry 2014. [Epub ahead of print].

44. Olaya JE, Christian E, Ferman D, et al. Deep brain stimulation in children and young adults with secondary dystonia: the Children's Hospital Los Angeles experience. Neurosurg Focus 2013;35(5):E7.

45. Gimeno H, Tustin K, Lumsden D, et al. Evaluation of functional goal outcomes using the Canadian Occupational Performance Measure (COPM) following deep brain stimulation (DBS) in childhood dystonia. Eur J Paediatr Neurol 2014;18:308–16.

Scoliosis, Spinal Fusion, and Intrathecal Baclofen Pump Implantation

 CrossMark

Brian Scannell, MD[a], Burt Yaszay, MD[b],*

KEYWORDS

- Scoliosis • Cerebral palsy • Spinal fusion • Intrathecal baclofen pump

KEY POINTS

- The incidence of scoliosis in patients with cerebral palsy is high, particularly in those with more involvement.
- Because of severe spasticity, many patients with cerebral palsy undergo intrathecal baclofen pump placement before, during, or after posterior spinal fusion.
- Despite high complications, it seems equally safe to place intrathecal baclofen pumps before, during, or after spinal fusion.

INTRODUCTION

Patients with cerebral palsy (CP) commonly develop scoliosis. The treatment of scoliosis in these patients can be different from treatment of the idiopathic scoliosis population. Management of the spinal deformity in CP can be challenging and often presents the surgeons and caregivers with many difficult decisions and obstacles. The approach to the care of these children should be multidisciplinary in order to optimize outcomes and decrease the frequent complications.

CEREBRAL PALSY AND SCOLIOSIS

The neuromuscular scoliosis that occurs in CP is typically a C-shaped curve that is often kyphoscoliotic and is associated with pelvic obliquity (**Fig. 1**). Children with CP have an increased risk of developing scoliosis compared with other patient populations.[1] Muscle weakness, truncal imbalance, and asymmetric tone in paraspinal muscles have long been implicated for the onset of scoliosis in CP, but there is little literature to support this theory.[2]

The authors have nothing to disclose.
[a] Department of Orthopaedics, Levine Children's Hospital, Carolinas Medical Center, 1001 Blythe Blvd, Suite 200, Charlotte, NC 28203, USA; [b] Department of Pediatric Orthopaedics, Rady Children's Hospital San Diego, 3020 Children's Way, San Diego, CA 92123, USA
* Corresponding author.
E-mail address: byaszay@rchsd.org

Phys Med Rehabil Clin N Am 26 (2015) 79–88
http://dx.doi.org/10.1016/j.pmr.2014.09.003
1047-9651/15/$ – see front matter © 2015 Elsevier Inc. All rights reserved.

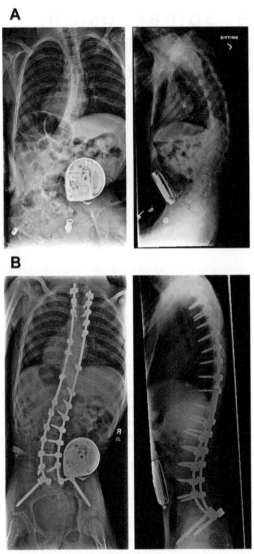

Fig. 1. (*A*) Anteroposterior/lateral radiographs of 14-year-old boy with scoliosis secondary to CP. The patient has undergone prior baclofen pump placement. (*B*) The patient has undergone correction of the scoliosis with a T2-pelvis fusion.

The prevalence of scoliosis in a total population of children with CP is nearly 30%.[3] Curves tend to begin at an earlier age than in idiopathic scoliosis.[4] They are more likely to progress even after the patient reaches skeletal maturity.[5] There is also an increased incidence of increased Gross Motor Function Classification System (GMFCS) level.[3] Children with GMFCS level IV and V CP have a 50% risk of moderate or severe scoliosis by the age of 18 years.[3]

Studies have found correlation between the size of the deformity and the decline in functional activities. Majd and colleagues[6] found an increased curve progression in patients with a decline in function compared with patients who were functionally stable. They also found that patients developing decubitus ulcers with prolonged sitting were more likely to have larger curves.

SCOLIOSIS TREATMENT IN CEREBRAL PALSY
Nonsurgical Treatment

Nonoperative treatment of scoliosis in patients with CP consists of:

- Observation
- Seating modifications
- Bracing

Observation can be chosen for curves of any size or magnitude. Reasons for continued observation are numerous. The curve size may be of insufficient magnitude to require surgical treatment. In addition, family decisions may be made to avoid operative management or other nonoperative modalities because of various comorbidities or after weighing the risks and benefits.

Molded wheelchair inserts can be used to attempt to improve overall sitting balance. Three-point force configuration support systems have been shown to achieve the best static correction of the scoliosis.[7] However, there is no evidence that this alters the natural history.[8] Modifications of the wheelchair should be individually tailored to the patient.

Bracing goals for CP are often different from the goals in idiopathic scoliosis. There is little evidence that bracing slows curve progression,[9] but there are many studies that show no significant effect of bracing.[10,11] The goals of bracing are to maintain comfortable, upright sitting, allow functional use of the upper extremities, and allow maximum ability to interact with the environment.[12] Soft braces seem to be tolerated better than rigid orthoses in patients with spastic CP. Soft braces maintain skin integrity[13] and potentially minimize respiratory compromise.[14]

Surgical Treatment

Goals, indications, and benefits of surgery, as well as the risk and potential complications, must be carefully weighed with the patient's family. There is no absolute indication of surgery (**Box 1**).[2,8,15]

For patients undergoing surgery, a thorough preoperative assessment is required. Assessment needs to include pulmonary function, nutritional status, gastrointestinal evaluation, and neurologic function.[2,8]

Pulmonary function testing is not easily performed in this patient population, but evaluation with a chest radiograph is often necessary. Patients with poor nutrition (serum albumin <35 g/L and total blood lymphocyte count <1.5 g/L) are known to have increased postoperative infection rate, longer length of intubation, and longer

---

Box 1
Goals of surgery and relative surgical indications for spinal fusion

Goals of Surgery	Relative Surgical Indications for Spinal Fusion
Improve coronal and sagittal balance	Progression of Cobb angle >50°
Improve sitting balance	Deterioration in functional sitting
Halt progression of scoliosis	Age >10 years, with adequate hip range of motion to
Level pelvis	allow seating, stable nutritional, and medical status
Improve positional discomfort	

hospital stays.[16] Nutrition may need to be optimized with nutritional supplementation or even a G-tube placement. From a gastrointestinal standpoint, assessment for gastroesophageal reflux and aspiration risk is needed because these patients are at risk for aspiration pneumonia.

In addition, seizure disorders should be controlled, and the medications used to control the condition should be noted. Some medications, such as phenytoin, phenobarbital, and valproic acid, can cause reduced bone mineral densities.[17] Valproic acid has also been implicated for increased intraoperative blood loss and the need for blood transfusions.[18]

The technical aspects of surgery for spinal fusion are beyond the scope of this article. There have been major advancements from a surgical standpoint from Luque rods, Luque rods with Galveston technique, unit rod fixation, Cotrel-Dubousset and Isola instrumentation, and more recently pedicle instrumentation. Pedicle instrumentation has been shown to have improved curve correction rates, lowest loss of correction, and greatest apical vertebral translation.[19]

The complication rate in the perioperative period for these patients is nearly 30%.[20] Patients with CP undergoing surgery for spinal deformity are at high risk for complications secondary to medical comorbidities.[8] Reames and colleagues[21] and Hod-Feins and colleagues[22] found surgical complications rates to be much higher among this patient population compared with the rates in idiopathic scoliosis. Perioperative complications including delayed extubation and length of hospital stay are significantly higher in neuromuscular scoliosis compared with idiopathic scoliosis.[22] This difference is likely directly related to longer surgeries, higher blood loss, and other medical comorbidities such as seizure disorders.[20,22]

Major complications in the postoperative period have also been described. Death is reported in 0% to 7% of patients.[23,24] Sponseller and colleagues[25] reported a deep infection rate of 6% and superficial rate of 4%. Deep infections in patients with CP are often polymicrobial with gram-negative organisms.[26] Pseudoarthrosis rates have decreased over time from the use of Harrington rods (as high as 40%) to Luque instrumentation (0%–13%) to more recent fixation with pedicle instrumentation (1%) **(Box 2)**.[26,27]

Outcomes of spinal fusion are difficult to assess in this patient population because there is still no adequate outcome tool to adequately assess improvement in function. Cassidy and colleagues[28] showed no clinically significant differences in pain, pulmonary medication need, decubitus ulcers, function, or time for daily care in patients who underwent spinal fusion compared with those who had not. In contrast, Larsson and colleagues[29] evaluated patients 1 year after surgery and found improvement in curve size and sitting balance. Multiple studies have shown high satisfaction in parents and

---

Box 2
Complications with spinal fusion in patients with CP

Perioperative Complications	Postoperative Complications
Death	Death
Neurologic complications	Superficial/deep infections
Respiratory distress, atelectasis, pneumonia	Pseudoarthrosis
Delayed extubation	Implant failure
Gastric distension, ileus, obstruction	
Seizures	
Blood loss	
Hemodynamic instability	

caregivers after surgery.[29–31] Based on a caregiver questionnaire, Watanabe and colleagues[31] found improvements in sitting balance (93%), cosmesis (94%), and quality of life (71%).

SCOLIOSIS, SPINAL FUSION, AND INTRATHECAL BACLOFEN PUMPS
Indications/Benefits of Intrathecal Baclofen Pumps

Intrathecal baclofen (ITB) is approved for treatment of spasticity related to several disorders including CP.[32] It inhibits both monosynaptic and polysynaptic reflexes at the spinal cord level thus decreasing excitatory neurotransmitter release from primary afferent terminals to decrease spasticity. Penn and Kroin[33] first reported its use for severe spasticity with immediate reduction of muscle tone to near-normal levels. The efficacy of ITB in children with CP is well documented.[34] Multiple studies have shown improvement in patients with CP. Gooch and colleagues[35] showed improved satisfaction of care providers, ease of care, and decreased pain. Other studies have also found improved ease of care[36] and others have shown improved gait in ambulatory patients with CP.[37] In addition, Gerszten and colleagues[37] showed a decreased need for subsequent orthopedic surgery for lower extremity spasticity. The indications for implantation of ITB pumps are primarily for intractable spasticity (**Box 3**).

Technique for Insertion of Intrathecal Baclofen Pumps

A trial test dose is frequently given before proceeding with placement of an ITB pump. This test can be performed on an inpatient or outpatient basis. Typical response is within 1 to 2 hours and lasts up to 8 hours. Based on this, it may be recommended to proceed with ITB pump implantation.

There are 2 components to the ITB pump infusion system: the pump, which commonly is implanted on the abdominal wall, and the catheter, which travels from the pump to the cerebrospinal fluid (CSF). Depending on the reservoir size and the dosing, the pump can hold enough drug for 4 to 6 months of therapy. It is refilled with a subcutaneous injection into the pump. Because many of these patients undergo spinal fusions, options for ITB pump placement include before, during, or after scoliosis surgery. Technical descriptions of placement are present in the literature.[8,38]

ITB pump placement before spinal fusion is technically less demanding than after spinal fusion. Patients are positioned in a lateral decubitus position. A midline incision is placed at the mid to lower lumbar level at the level of the iliac crest. This placement can easily be incorporated into any future incision needed for a spinal fusion. A separate fascial incision is made approximately 1 cm lateral from midline. The catheter is placed below the fascia to provide an additional layer of closure. A 14-gauge Tuohy needle is directed midline and obliquely in a cephalad direction so as to be placed

---

Box 3	
Indications for ITB pump and benefits of ITB pump therapy	
Indications for ITB Pump Therapy	**Benefits of ITB Pump Therapy**
Intractable spasticity	Improved spasticity
Uncontrollable spasticity with drug therapy	Improved range of motion
Intolerable side effects to oral baclofen	Improved ease of care
	Improved pain
	Increased caregiver satisfaction
	Improved hygiene, transfers
	Improved gait

into the dural sac between L2/3 or L3/4. Fluoroscopy is used to confirm intrathecal placement and to guide advancement to the appropriate level. The final catheter placement is guided by diagnosis, the extremities affected, and the desired effect.[8] Most pumps are placed on the right side to avoid current or future gastrostomy tubes. An incision is made in this location and a subcutaneous or subfascial pocket is developed in order to place the pump. In thin patients with CP, the pump is typically placed subfascially to ensure an additional layer of closure. The subfascial placement of the catheter and pump provide an additional barrier to CSF leak, which can complicate the procedure.[39] The catheter is then tunneled from the spine to the pump and is tested to ensure backflow of CSF.

When placing the ITB pump after a spinal fusion, an incision is made through the previous midline scar and a subperiosteal exposure of the fusion mass is performed.[38] Fluoroscopy is used to locate the implants and the level of spine exposed. The technique of using a burr to open a hole in the fusion mass at L2/3 or L3/4 has been described.[38] If a large hole is made, this increases the risk of CSF leak. This risk can be minimized by leaving a thin layer of bone and pushing the Tuohy needle through it to gain access to the spinal canal. At our institution (Rady Children's Hospital San Diego) we have modified this technique depending on the type of spinal instrumentation used. In cases in which sublaminar wires have been used, the wires at L3 or L4 are removed. This hole in the fusion mass left by the wire is typically large enough for the catheter needle to enter the spinal canal. In patients instrumented with segmental pedicle screws, a 2-mm K-wire is used to create an oblique hole through the lower lumbar fusion mass. Under fluoroscopic guidance, the K-wire is oscillated through the fusion mass. Tactile feedback typically shows when the spinal canal is entered. In many cases, the K-wire has not punctured the thecal sac. Once the catheter is placed and secured similarly to that described earlier, bone wax and/or fibrin sealant is placed around the fusion mass hole to minimize the risk of CSF leak.

Patients with prior ITB pump implantation who undergo a posterior spinal fusion (PSF) can be approached in several ways. It is possible to work around the catheter and keep it intact, although this can be frustrating to the surgeon. The catheter can be removed and the dura can be sealed uneventfully with a new catheter placed after spinal fusion. It is also possible to cut the current catheter and then reanastomose with some systems.

Complications of Intrathecal Baclofen Pump Placement

Although the safety and efficacy of ITB pumps has been evaluated,[34,35,37] there are still significant complications associated with their placement before, during, or after spinal fusion in patients with CP. Complications related to ITB pump placement are well reported in the pediatric literature (**Box 4**).[39–44]

Wound complications and infections are also a common reason for rehospitalization and reoperation in patients with CP. Fjelstad and colleagues[43] found the rate of infection after ITB pumpplacement to be higher in children than in adults (10% vs 0%), but more of the pediatric patients had a diagnosis of CP compared with the adult population in this study. Overall acute infection rates ranged from 4% to 10%.[39,42] One study found a significant increase in infection rate with subcutaneous pump placement compared with subfascial placement (20.1% vs 3.6%; $P<.001$) and thus recommended subfascial placement.[39] When infection occurs, there is a high rate of reoperation and removal of the catheter and pump.[40,44]

The incidences of catheter-related and pump-related complications are variable in the literature. Complications include pump malfunction and catheter dislodgement/breakage/malfunction. Rippe and colleagues[41] reported a total of 264 catheter

---

Box 4
Perioperative and postoperative complications of ITB pumps

Perioperative Complications of ITB Pumps	Postoperative Complications of ITB Pumps
Bleeding	CSF leak
CSF leak	Infection: pump, CSF
Initial alteration in bladder control	Wound dehiscence
Apnea, respiratory depression	Catheter-related complications: catheter
Baclofen overdose: lethargy, seizures,	breakage/dislodgement/malfunction
respiratory depression	Pump failure
	Seroma at pump site
	Risk of scoliosis progression
	Need for reoperation for one of the
	complications listed earlier

---

complications in 785 patients. Borowoski and colleagues[42] reported 16% to 27% device complications in their patients, most which were catheter malfunctions. Armstrong and colleagues[36] reported 10 complications in 19 patients over 568 months. Similar to infections, the complications related to catheters and pumps are a common reason for rehospitalization and reoperation.[45]

An additional complication reported with ITB pump placement before scoliosis surgery is progression of scoliosis. Significant controversy exists as to whether insertion of ITB pumps causes progression of scoliosis in patients with CP,[46–52] and some clinicians think that the progression is related to patients who receive an ITB pump being more severely involved and thus their natural history is to have progressive scoliosis.[8]

Two series of patients reported accelerated scoliosis progression after ITB pump placement.[47,48] Segal and colleagues[47] initially presented their series of 5 patients with a mean progression of 44° over 11 months leading to spinal fusion. Burn and colleagues[50] found an annual progression of Cobb angle of 18° and an increase in progression per year in patients less than 15 years old at the time of ITB pump placement. Ginsburg and Lauder[46] found an increase in scoliosis progression from 1.8°/y before implantation to 10.9°/y after implantation.

However, these studies supporting progression of scoliosis after ITB pump placement were small series. In contrast, 2 studies that compared matched cohorts of patients with CP with and without ITB pumps found no difference in the rate of scoliosis progression.[51,52] In the study by Shilt and colleagues,[52] patients were matched by diagnosis of CP, age, sex, topographic involvement, and initial Cobb angle. No difference was found between the mean change in Cobb angle in the patients with ITB pumps (6.6° per year) compared with the controls (5.0° per year).

In addition, there is also concern and debate about whether prior placement of an ITB pump can further complicate CP scoliosis surgery and increase the risk for wound complications. There are 2 studies that have compared the outcomes of PSF in CP with and without ITB pumps.[38,45] Caird and colleagues[45] compared 20 patients with spastic quadriplegic CP with ITB pump who underwent PSF with 20 matched patients without an ITB pump. They found increased reoperation and rehospitalization, as mentioned previously, and a higher infection rate in the ITB pump group (20% vs 0%; $P = .063$). However, the patients in the ITB pump group had more preoperative comorbidities.

Borowski and colleagues[38] compared 4 groups of patients with CP: PSF before ITB pump placement (n=26), PSF and ITB pump placement concurrently (n=11), PSF after ITB pump placement (n=25), and ITB pump placement only (n=103). In all four groups, they found an infection rate of 8% to 9% with no differences between groups. There was also no difference in device or catheter complications between groups. They concluded that ITB pumps are able to be implanted and managed without any increase in complication rate before, during, or after spinal fusion.

SUMMARY

The incidence of scoliosis in patients with CP is high, particularly in those with more involvement. Many of these patients undergo spinal fusion for the scoliosis. However, complication rates are extremely high. The risks and benefits must be thoroughly discussed with the patient's family and caregiver before proceeding with surgery. Because of severe spasticity, many of these patients undergo ITB pump placement before, during, or after PSF. The complication rates are high with ITB pump placement, but many patients have significant benefit. Despite high complications, it seems equally safe to place ITB pumps before, during, or after spinal fusion.

REFERENCES

1. Madigan RR, Wallace SL. Scoliosis in the institutionalized cerebral palsy population. Spine 1981;6:583–90.
2. McCarthy J, D'Andrea L, Betz R, et al. Scoliosis in the child with cerebral palsy. J Am Acad Orthop Surg 2006;14(6):367–75.
3. Persson-Bunke M, Hagglund G, Lauge-Pederson H, et al. Scoliosis in a total population of children with cerebral palsy. Spine 2012;37:E708–13.
4. Saito N, Ebara S, Ohotsuka K, et al. Natural history of scoliosis in spastic cerebral palsy. Lancet 1998;351:1687–92.
5. Thometz JG, Simon SR. Progression of scoliosis after skeletal maturity in institutionalized adults who have cerebral palsy. J Bone Joint Surg 1988;70:1290–6.
6. Majd M, Muldowny D, Holt R. Natural history of scoliosis in the institutionalized adult cerebral palsy population. Spine 1997;22:1461–6.
7. Holmes K, Michael S, Thorpe S, et al. Management of scoliosis with special seating for the nonambulant spastic cerebral palsy population - a biomechanical study. Clin Biomech 2003;18(6):480–7.
8. Imrie M, Yaszay B. Management of spinal deformity in cerebral palsy. Orthop Clin North Am 2010;41:531–47.
9. Terjesen T, Lange J, Steen H. Treatment of scoliosis with spinal bracing in quadriplegic Cerebral Palsy. Dev Med Child Neurol 2000;42:448–54.
10. Miller A, Temple T, Miller F. Impact of orthoses on the rate of scoliosis progression in children with cerebral palsy. J Pediatr Orthop 1996;16:332–5.
11. Renshaw T, Green N, Griffin PP, et al. Cerebral palsy: orthopaedic management. Instr Course Lect 1996;45:475–90.
12. Rutz E, Brunner R. Management of spinal deformity in cerebral palsy: conservative treatment. J Child Orthop 2013;7:415–8.
13. Letts M, Rathbone D, Yamashita T, et al. Soft Boston Orthosis management of neuromuscular scoliosis: a preliminary report. J Pediatr Orthop 1992;12:470–4.
14. Leopando M, Moussavi Z, Holbrow J, et al. Effect of a soft Boston Orthosis on pulmonary mechanics in severe cerebral palsy. Pediatr Pulmonol 1999;28:53–8.
15. Hasler C. Operative treatment for spinal deformities in cerebral palsy. J Child Orthop 2013;7:419–23.

16. Jevsevar D, Karlin L. The relationship between preoperative nutritional status and complications after an operation for scoliosis in patients who have cerebral palsy. J Bone Joint Surg Am 1993;75:880–4.
17. Farhat F, Yamout B, Mikati M. Effect of antiepileptic drugs on bone density in ambulatory patients. Neurology 2002;58:1348–53.
18. Chambers H, Weinstein C, Mubarak S, et al. The effect of valproic acid on blood loss in patients with cerebral palsy. J Pediatr Orthop 1999;19:792–5.
19. Watanabe K, Lenke L, Bridwell K, et al. Comparison of radiographic outcomes for the treatment of scoliotic curves greater than 100 degrees: wires versus hooks versus screws. Spine 2008;33:1084–92.
20. Mohamad F, Parent S, Pawelek J, et al. Perioperative complications after surgical correction in neuromuscular scoliosis. J Pediatr Orthop 2007;27(4):392–7.
21. Reames D, Smith J, Fu K, et al. Complications in the surgical treatment of 19,360 cases of pediatric scoliosis: a review of the Scoliosis Research Society Database. Spine 2011;36(18):1484–91.
22. Hod-Feins R, Abu-Kishk I, Eshel G, et al. Risk factors affecting the immediate post-operative course in pediatric scoliosis surgery. Spine (Phila Pa 1976) 2007;32(21):2355–60.
23. Broom M, Banta J, Renshaw T. Spinal fusion augmented by Luque-rod segmental instrumentation for neuromuscular scoliosis. J Bone Joint Surg Am 1989;71:32–44.
24. Sarwark J, Sarwarhi V. New strategies and decision making in the management of neuromuscular scoliosis. Orthop Clin North Am 2007;38:485–96.
25. Sponseller P, LaPorte D, Hungerford M, et al. Infection rate after spine surgery in cerebral palsy is high and impairs results: multicenter analysis of risk factors and treatment. Clin Orthop Relat Res 2010;468:711–6.
26. Newton P, Capelo R. Spinal deformity in cerebral palsy. In: Kim D, Betz R, Huhn S, et al, editors. Surgery of the pediatric spine. New York: Thieme Medical Publishers, Inc; 2008. p. 441–56.
27. Tsirikos A, Lipton G, Chang W, et al. Surgical correction of scoliosis in pediatric patients with cerebral palsy using the unit rod instrumentation. Spine 2008;33:1133–40.
28. Cassidy C, Craig C, Perry A, et al. A reassessment of spinal stabilization in severe cerebral palsy. J Pediatr Orthop 1994;12:731–9.
29. Larsson E, Aaro S, Oberg B. Activities and functional assessment 1 year after spinal fusion for paralytic scoliosis. Eur Spine J 1999;8:100–9.
30. Tsirikos A, Chang W, Dabney K, et al. Comparison of parents' and caregivers' satisfaction after spinal fusion in children with cerebral palsy. J Pediatr Orthop 2004;24:54–8.
31. Watanabe K, Lenke L, Daubs M, et al. Is spine deformity surgery in patients with spastic cerebral palsy truly beneficial? A patient/parent evaluation. Spine 2009;34:2222–32.
32. Lynn AK, Turner M, Chambers HG. Surgical management of spasticity in persons with cerebral palsy. PM R 2009;1(9):834–8.
33. Penn RD, Kroin JS. Continuous intrathecal baclofen for severe spasticity. Lancet 1985;2(8447):125–7.
34. Albright AL, Cervi A, Singletary J. Intrathecal baclofen for spasticity in cerebral palsy. JAMA 1991;265(11):1418–22.
35. Gooch JL, Oberg WA, Grams B, et al. Care provider assessment of intrathecal baclofen in children. Dev Med Child Neurol 2004;46(8):548–52.
36. Armstrong RW, Steinbok P, Cochrane DD, et al. Intrathecally administered baclofen for treatment of children with spasticity of cerebral origin. J Neurosurg 1997;87(3):409–14.

37. Gerszten PC, Albright AL, Johnstone GF. Intrathecal baclofen infusion and subsequent orthopedic surgery in patients with spastic cerebral palsy. J Neurosurg 1998;88(6):1009–13.

38. Borowski A, Shah SA, Littleton AG, et al. Baclofen pump implantation and spinal fusion in children: techniques and complications. Spine (Phila Pa 1976) 2008; 33(18):1995–2000.

39. Motta F, Antonello P. Analysis of complications in 430 consecutive pediatric patients treated with intrathecal baclofen therapy: 14-year experience. J Neurosurg Pediatr 2014;13:301–6.

40. Dickey MP, Rice M, Kinnett DG, et al. Infectious complications of intrathecal baclofen pump devices in a pediatric population. Pediatr Infect Dis J 2013;32(7): 715–22.

41. Rippe D, Tann B, Gaebler-Spira D, et al. Complications of intrathecal baclofen pump therapy for severe hypertonia in children: a long-term follow-up review of 785 patients from four centers. Dev Med Child Neurol 2005;47(suppl 102):14.

42. Borowski A, Littleton AG, Borkhuu B, et al. Complications of intrathecal baclofen pump therapy in pediatric patients. J Pediatr Orthop 2010;30(1):76–81.

43. Fjelstad AB, Hommelstad J, Sorteberg A. Infections related to intrathecal baclofen therapy in children and adults: frequency and risk factors. J Neurosurg Pediatr 2009;4(5):487–93.

44. Murphy NA, Irwin MC, Hoff C. Intrathecal baclofen therapy in children with cerebral palsy: efficacy and complications. Arch Phys Med Rehabil 2002;83(12): 1721–5.

45. Caird MS, Palanca AA, Garton H, et al. Outcomes of posterior spinal fusion and instrumentation in patients with continuous intrathecal baclofen infusion pumps. Spine (Phila Pa 1976) 2008;33(4):E94–9.

46. Ginsburg GM, Lauder AJ. Progression of scoliosis in patients with spastic quadriplegia after the insertion of an intrathecal baclofen pump. Spine (Phila Pa 1976) 2007;32(24):2745–50.

47. Segal LS, Wallach DM, Kanev PM. Potential complications of posterior spine fusion and instrumentation in patients with cerebral palsy treated with intrathecal baclofen infusion. Spine (Phila Pa 1976) 2005;30(8):E219–24.

48. Sansone JM, Mann D, Noonan K, et al. Rapid progression of scoliosis following insertion of intrathecal baclofen pump. J Pediatr Orthop 2006;26(1):125–8.

49. Krach LE, Walker K, Rapp L. The effect of intrathecal baclofen treatment on the development of scoliosis in individuals with cerebral palsy: a retrospective case-matched review. Dev Med Child Neurol 2005;47(suppl 102):14.

50. Burn SC, Zeller R, Drake JM. Do baclofen pumps influence the development of scoliosis in children? J Neurosurg Pediatr 2010;5(2):195–9.

51. Senaran H, Shah SA, Presedo A, et al. The risk of progression of scoliosis in cerebral palsy patients after intrathecal baclofen therapy. Spine (Phila Pa 1976) 2007;32(21):2348–54.

52. Shilt JS, Lai LP, Cabrera MN, et al. The impact of intrathecal baclofen on the natural history of scoliosis in cerebral palsy. J Pediatr Orthop 2008;28(6):684–7.

Intrathecal Baclofen Bolus Dosing and Catheter Tip Placement in Pediatric Tone Management

Andrew J. Skalsky, MD[a],*, Chrystal M. Fournier, MSN, RN, FNP-BC[b]

KEYWORDS

- Pediatric • Cerebral palsy • Intrathecal baclofen • Spasticity • Flex • Bolus
- Catheter

KEY POINTS

- High cervical catheter tip placement in intrathecal baclofen (ITB) therapy may be more efficacious.
- Pulsating, bolus, or flex dosing of ITB may be more efficacious than simple continuous infusion.
- There is a large concentration gradient within the cerebral spinal fluid (CSF).
- CSF flow oscillates along a craniocaudal axis and is not a continuous mixing flow as once portrayed.

INTRODUCTION

Nature of the Problem

Intrathecal baclofen (ITB) administered by an implanted pump was approved by the US Food and Drug Administration for the treatment of spasticity of cerebral origin in 1996. Intrathecal baclofen results in fewer systemic side effects than enteral baclofen with higher efficacy. Regarding cerebral palsy, efficacy evidence for managing spasticity was first published in 2000.[1] There has been increasing evidence that ITB is an efficacious treatment for spasticity in children.[2] Most of the studies assessing efficacy are based on a simple continuous infusion of ITB and little is mentioned regarding daily dosing or catheter tip placement.[3,4]

Disclosure: The authors have nothing to disclose.
[a] Division of Pediatric Rehabilitation Medicine, Department of Pediatrics, Rady Children's Hospital San Diego, University of California San Diego, 3020 Children's Way MC 5096, San Diego, CA 92123, USA; [b] Division of Pediatric Rehabilitation Medicine, Rady Children's Hospital San Diego, 3020 Children's Way, San Diego, CA 92123, USA
* Corresponding author.
E-mail address: askalsky@rchsd.org

Phys Med Rehabil Clin N Am 26 (2015) 89–93
http://dx.doi.org/10.1016/j.pmr.2014.09.011
1047-9651/15/$ – see front matter © 2015 Elsevier Inc. All rights reserved.

Overall, patient satisfaction with intrathecal baclofen is high.[5] Krach and colleagues[6] showed that intrathecal baclofen therapy does not adversely affect the mortality of patients receiving this therapeutic modality compared with a matched cohort. One retrospective review found that after 1 year of ITB treatment, the mean ITB dose when treating spasticity was approximately 300 μg per day.[7] Despite more than 20 years of clinical use of ITB, there are several unanswered questions, including the ideal catheter tip placement and dosing regimens.

Pulsatile Dosing

Progressive dose increases are thought to be caused by tolerance, defined as requiring a higher dose to achieve the same degree of desired effect. Most practitioners experience this soon after a new ITB pump is implanted. Many patients are well controlled on relatively low doses soon after implantation, but the magnitude of effect quickly dissipates, requiring dose escalation.[8] Pulsatile bolus doses have been proposed as an effective and safe treatment strategy to reverse the need for increasing ITB dosages in patients with the probable tolerance to ITB.[9] There is a paucity of reports regarding ITB dosing regimens as alternative to simple continuous infusion. The published reports have been retrospective case series.[10,11] Interestingly, most clinicians reserve flex or bolus dosing for more severe cases or cases of primarily dystonia that were relatively unresponsive to simple continuous ITB therapy. This supports the notion that pulsatile bolus dosing of ITB may be more efficacious. No studies have compared the efficacy of simple continuous infusion to pulsatile bolus dosing.

Catheter Tip Location

There is one report reviewing the association of catheter tip location and daily dosing. The catheter tip location was variable because no intraoperative imaging was used to determine the catheter tip location. There was a trend for the higher catheter tip placement, resulting in lower daily doses (**Table 1**); however, "linear regression showed that a higher-level intrathecal catheter needs a lower dose, but this was not significant."[12]

Theory Behind Catheter Tip Location and Pulsatile Dosing

We know there is a significant concentration gradient that develops in the cerebral spinal fluid (CSF) for almost all naturally occurring proteins, neurotransmitters, and metabolites.[13,14] The exact mechanism of this is unknown. There is also a concentration gradient for ITB. Bernards[15] demonstrated that the concentration of baclofen is only 0.5% at a distance of 5 cm in comparison with the catheter tip at a steady state with a continuous low dose infusion. This was dramatically increased to almost 50%

Table 1
The number of cases with the intrathecal catheter tips at each level in the spine, along with the mean dose

Level	Number	Mean Dose (μg/d)	SE
Cervical	9	197.8	±78.1
Thoracic	81	266.2	±23.4
Lumbar	15	228.6	±49.5
Sacral	3	466.7	±280.4

Adapted from Sivakumar G, Yap Y, Tsegaye M, et al. Intrathecal baclofen therapy for spasticity of cerebral origin—does the position of the intrathecal catheter matter? Childs Nerv Syst 2010;26(8):1097–102. PMID: 20306056.

with a high-dose continuous infusion. However, this was increased even further when a single large bolus was administered. The large bolus raised the concentration at 5 cm to within 75% of the catheter tip and was still 23% at 10 cm. At either continuous infusion rate, the concentration at 10 cm was virtually undetectable. It is hypothesized by the author that the source of energy to facilitate the greater drug distribution within the CSF is the kinetic energy imparted to the drug by the act of the injection. The drug infusion in a simple continuous infusion is almost imperceptible. The faster infusion and especially the bolus imparts a slight, but observable, forward motion to the injectate, and differences among the drug distributions may be in part the result of differences in kinetic energy associated with the different infusion rates.[15]

In addition to concentration gradients within the CSF, it has been demonstrated that the CSF flow oscillates along a craniocaudal axis. There is not a continuous mixing flow caudad along the posterior surface of the spinal cord and returning cephalad along the anterior surface as if it were a river, which was once portrayed. Enzmann and Pelc[16] showed that the flow velocity is greatest in the cervical spine and is essentially absent in the distal lumbar sac. The higher flow velocities in the cervical spine in comparison with the lumbar spine may help disperse the ITB over a larger area. The higher CSF flow should result in a lower concentration gradient over a longer spinal segment in the cervical spine in comparison with the lumbar region. The lack of CSF flow in the lumbosacral spine also may explain why the patients with sacral catheter tip placements required more than double the dose in comparison with the patients with a cervical catheter tip.[12]

Many practitioners note a decrease in efficacy when changing to a higher concentration of ITB despite no change in the actual daily dose. The higher concentration results in a lower volume infusion, which is accompanied by less kinetic energy. The previously described mechanism of kinetic energy may account for this difference in therapeutic effect.

Case Report Demonstration of Theory

A 15-year-old boy with Gross Motor Function Classification System IV spastic quadriparetic cerebral palsy underwent implantation of an ITB pump. In the early postoperative period, his dose was titrated to 350 μg per day using a simple continuous infusion. His delivery method was changed from simple continuous infusion to a flex dosing regimen with bolus administration every 4 hours. Because the pump being used (Synchromed II; Medtronic, Minneapolis, MN) has a minimum basal rate of 0.002 mL per hour or 4 μg per hour when using a 2000 μg/mL concentration, the 4-hour bolus dose was programmed to be 40 μg, which made the total daily dosage 335 μg, a 4.3% reduction in total daily dosing. Within 12 hours, he had clear symptoms of overdose with nausea, vomiting, lethargy, and confusion but unchanged heart rate, blood pressure, respiratory rate, and pulse oximetry measurements. The bolus dose was decreased by an additional 25% to 30 μg every 4 hours with a resulting total daily dosage of 275 μg. Over the next 12 hours, there was complete resolution of the overdose symptoms and the resulting tone management was comparable to the original 350-μg simple continuous infusion despite a more than 20% reduction in the total daily dosage.

Postimplantation Titration

An additional advantage of pulsatile bolus dosing in comparison with simple continuous infusions is that it allows for a more rapid initial titration of the dose. Because sudden large dose changes are typically not well tolerated, the dose escalation with a simple continuous infusion is a relatively slow process with increases of 10% to 20% per adjustment. With a bolus administration schedule, each bolus can be progressively larger, resulting in a relatively high daily dose increase that is generally well tolerated because it is a small dose increase every 3 to 4 hours in comparison with the total daily dosage. The pump must be reprogrammed within 24 hours or the bolus dose will drop back down to initial dose and benefit of the dose escalation will be lost. A typical postimplantation titration is included in **Box 1** starting with postoperative day 1. The functional total daily dosage can be increased by 102% within 48 hours. This large of an increase in a simple continuous infusion would place the patient at a high risk for overdose.

Our Experience

More than 90% of the patients at our institution with an ITB pump have changed to a bolus dosing regimen with a higher rate of satisfaction in comparison with simple continuous infusions. We have trialed different bolus intervals, with most patients experiencing a cyclical effect with boluses spaced more than 4 hours apart. A small percentage of patients with primarily dystonia require more frequent boluses every 3 hours to prevent a cyclic response to the therapy.

Box 1
Example of rapid dose escalation while using pulsatile or bolus dosing

Postoperative Day 1		
Start Time (h:min)	**Dose (μg)**	**Duration (h:min)**
Monday–Sunday		
Basal Rate 4.00 μg/h		
00:00	4.00	00:05
04:00	5.00	00:05
08:00	6.00	00:05
12:00	1.00	00:05
16:00	2.00	00:05
20:00	3.00	00:05
Total 114.86 μg/d		
Postoperative Day 2		
Start Time (h:min)	**Dose (μg)**	**Duration (h:min)**
Monday–Sunday		
Basal Rate 4.00 μg/h		
00:00	10.00	00:05
04:00	11.00	00:05
08:00	12.00	00:05
12:00	7.00	00:05
16:00	8.00	00:05
20:00	9.00	00:05
Total 149.93 μg/d		
Postoperative Day 3		
Start Time (h:min)	**Dose (μg)**	**Duration (h:min)**
Monday–Sunday		
Basal Rate 4.00 μg/h		
00:00	16.00	00:05
04:00	17.00	00:05
08:00	18.00	00:05
12:00	13.00	00:05
16:00	14.00	00:05
20:00	15.00	00:05
Total 186.87 μg/d		

REFERENCES

1. Butler C, Campbell S. Evidence of the effects of intrathecal baclofen for spastic and dystonic cerebral palsy. AACPDM Treatment Outcomes Committee Review Panel. Dev Med Child Neurol 2000;42:634–45.

2. Dan B, Motta F, Vles JS, et al. Consensus on the appropriate use of intrathecal baclofen (ITB) therapy in paediatric spasticity. Eur J Paediatr Neurol 2010; 14(1):19–28 Review. PMID: 19541514.

3. Morton RE, Gray N, Vloeberghs M. Controlled study of the effects of continuous intrathecal baclofen infusion in non-ambulant children with cerebral palsy. Dev Med Child Neurol 2011;53(8):736–41. PMID: 21707598.

4. Ramstad K, Jahnsen R, Lofterod B, et al. Continuous intrathecal baclofen therapy in children with cerebral palsy—when does improvement emerge? Acta Paediatr 2010;99(11):1661–5. PMID: 19912148.

5. Krach LE, Nettleton A, Klempka B. Satisfaction of individuals treated long-term with continuous infusion of intrathecal baclofen by implanted programmable pump. Pediatr Rehabil 2006;9:210–8.

6. Krach LE, Kriel RL, Day SM, et al. Survival of individuals with cerebral palsy receiving continuous intrathecal baclofen treatment: a case–control study. Dev Med Child Neurol 2010;52:672–6.

7. Albright AL, Gilmartin R, Swift D, et al. Long-term intrathecal baclofen therapy for severe spasticity of cerebral origin. J Neurosurg 2003;98:291–5.

8. Heetla HW, Staal MJ, Kliphuis C, et al. The incidence and management of tolerance in intrathecal baclofen therapy. Spinal Cord 2009;47:751–6.

9. Heetla HW, Staal MJ, van Laar T. Tolerance to continuous intrathecal baclofen infusion can be reversed by pulsatile bolus infusion. Spinal Cord 2010;48(6): 483–6. http://dx.doi.org/10.1038/sc.2009.156. PMID: 19918253.

10. Saval A, Chiodo AE. Intrathecal baclofen for spasticity management: a comparative analysis of spasticity of spinal vs cortical origin. J Spinal Cord Med 2010; 33(1):16–21. PMID: 20397440.

11. Krach LE, Kriel RL, Nugent AC. Complex dosing schedules for continuous intrathecal baclofen infusion. Pediatr Neurol 2007;37(5):354–9. PubMed PMID: 17950422.

12. Sivakumar G, Yap Y, Tsegaye M, et al. Intrathecal baclofen therapy for spasticity of cerebral origin–does the position of the intrathecal catheter matter? Childs Nerv Syst 2010;26(8):1097–102. PMID: 20306056.

13. Degrell I, Nagy E. Concentration gradients for HVA, 5-HIAA, ascorbic acid, and uric acid in cerebrospinal fluid. Biol Psychiatry 1990;27(8):891–6. PubMed PMID: 1691925.

14. Weisner B, Bernhardt W. Protein fractions of lumbar, cisternal, and ventricular cerebrospinal fluid. Separate areas of reference. J Neurol Sci 1978;37(3): 205–14. PMID: 681976.

15. Bernards CM. Cerebrospinal fluid and spinal cord distribution of baclofen and bupivacaine during slow intrathecal infusion in pigs. Anesthesiology 2006; 105(1):169–78. PMID: 16810009.

16. Enzmann DR, Pelc NJ. Normal flow patterns of intracranial and spinal cerebrospinal fluid defined with phase-contrast cine MR imaging. Radiology 1991;178(2): 467–74. PMID: 1987610.

Pediatric Limb Differences and Amputations

Joan T. Le, MD[a],*, Phoebe R. Scott-Wyard, DO[b,c]

KEYWORDS

- Pediatric limb difference • Congenital limb deficiency • Amputation

KEY POINTS

- Congenital limb differences are uncommon and often go undetected until birth.
- A thorough history, physical examination, or diagnostic workup should be done for children with congenital limb differences to rule out syndromes involving other organ systems or known associations.
- Acquired amputations most commonly occur from trauma.
- Complications, such as pain and terminal bony overgrowth can occur after amputation.
- A multidisciplinary approach to management is recommended, when available.

NATURE OF THE PROBLEM

The Centers for Disease Control and Prevention estimate that each year 2250 babies are born with congenital upper and/or lower limb deficiencies or reductions each year in the United States. This is approximately 6 per 10,000 live births per year, in a ratio of 2:1 upper to lower extremity.[1] Precise numbers for other forms of congenital limb differences (ie, limb length discrepancies, neuromuscular pathology leading to differences in limb) and joint deformities (ie, contractures) are not known. Recent data suggest a relationship between paternal occupation and increased prevalence of birth defects, including limb deficiencies, in offspring of artists.[2] No racial predilection has been noted. Medications known to affect limb development include thalidomide, retinoic acid, and misoprostol. Teratogenic causes are often challenging to discern, as prenatal history may be complicated by maternal recall bias, and the timing of limb development is coincident when the mother may not know she is pregnant.[3] Limb deficiencies can also be caused by vascular disruption (eg, amniotic band syndrome),

Disclosure: The authors have nothing to disclose.
[a] Division of Pediatric Rehabilitation Medicine, Department of Pediatrics, Rady Children's Hospital San Diego, University of California San Diego, 3020 Children's Way, MC 5096, San Diego, CA 92123, USA; [b] Child Amputee Prosthetics Project, Shriners Hospital - Los Angeles, 3160 Geneva St., Los Angeles, CA 90020, USA; [c] Pediatric Rehabilitation Division, Children's Hospital Los Angeles, 4650 Sunset Blvd., Los Angeles, CA 90027, USA
* Corresponding author.
E-mail address: joanle@rchsd.org

Phys Med Rehabil Clin N Am 26 (2015) 95–108
http://dx.doi.org/10.1016/j.pmr.2014.09.006
1047-9651/15/$ – see front matter © 2015 Elsevier Inc. All rights reserved.

pmr.theclinics.com

vascular malformations (eg, Poland syndrome), or genetic factors (spontaneous point mutation). Findings from experimental animal studies suggest that limb deficiency in amniotic band syndrome may be caused by a cascade of hypoxia, cell damage, hemorrhage, tissue loss, and reperfusion.[4] In most cases the cause is unknown.[5]

Acquired amputations most commonly occur from trauma or disease (ie, neoplasm or infection.) A retrospective study done in the United States determined that there were more than 110,000 children younger than 18 years that presented to emergency rooms with traumatic amputation injuries during a 12-year period. The average age was 6.18 years, patients were predominantly males (65.5%), and finger amputations comprised 91.6% of the amputations.[6]

Despite prenatal screening ultrasound scans, congenital limb deficiencies may not be detected before birth. The International Organization for Standardization (ISO) names congenital limb deficiencies as follows: transverse (normal limb development to a particular level, with no skeletal elements distally) and longitudinal (absence or reduction of an element within the long axis).[7]

Terminology used to differentiate acquired amputations in the upper limb includes shoulder disarticulation, transhumeral, elbow disarticulation, transradial, wrist disarticulation, and partial hand amputation. The different forms of lower limb amputations are translumbar, transpelvic, hip disarticulation, transfemoral, knee disarticulation, transtibial, ankle disarticulation, and partial foot amputation.[8]

PATHOPHYSIOLOGY

Limb development occurs between 4 and 8 weeks after fertilization. Most limb defects are thought to occur during weeks 4 and 6, during times of rapid tissue proliferation.[9] Limb development is considered with respect to its 3 axes of growth (proximal-distal, anterior-posterior/radio-ulnar, and dorsal-ventral.) Each axis is controlled by distinct, yet coordinated, molecular pathways, which include fibroblast growth factors, sonic hedgehog, and the Wingless-type signaling pathways. Each pathway is responsible for its own differentiation, yet they work in concert and have complex interactions with signaling, regulation, feedback loops, and maintenance of the other axes and embryogenesis. Errors in these pathways can indirectly affect the appropriate operation of other signaling centers, which may reflect the presence of other organ systems involved in some children with limb deficiencies.[10]

CONGENITAL LIMB DIFFERENCES
Upper Limb

Polydactyly is a congenital hand difference resulting in an extra digit. The extra digit may be preaxial (radially located) postaxial (ulnarly located) or centrally located. Most cases of preaxial polydactyly are sporadic and occur unilaterally. However, if the extra thumb has 3 phalanges, it may be linked to a systemic syndrome, such as Holt-Oram syndrome or Fanconi anemia. Postaxial polydactyly is often found in patients of African or African-American descent and can be inherited in an autosomal dominant pattern. If the postaxial digit is found in a Caucasian patient, there may be an underlying syndrome, such as chondroectodermal dysplasia or Ellis-van Creveld syndrome.

Syndactyly is a condition in which the digits fail to separate into individual appendages. Syndactyly can be simple, in which only the soft tissues are involved, or it can be complex, in which the bone or nail of the neighboring fingers is involved. It is typically an isolated finding; however, it may be associated with certain syndromes, such as Apert or Poland syndrome. Apert syndrome, or acrocephalosyndactyly, is characterized by complex syndactyly, craniosynostosis, hypertelorism, exophthalmos, and mild mental retardation.[11]

Amniotic constriction band, constriction band syndrome, or amniotic band syndrome can result in clinical manifestations including congenital limb differences, joint deformities, defects of the abdomen or chest wall, or craniofacial defects. Limb differences from amniotic band syndrome include digit or limb amputations, constriction rings, or acrosyndactyly. Multiple limbs can be involved, with greater involvement of the upper limb, especially the distal aspects and central digits. Because of the constriction, lymphedema can occur.

Transverse deficiencies of the upper limb can occur at any level. Partial hand deficiencies may have ipsilateral shortening of the radius and ulna with underdeveloped vestigial digits, often called nubbins. The most common transverse deficiency of the forearm occurs in the upper third, and children often have ipsilateral shortening of the humerus (**Figs. 1** and **2**). In those with transverse deficiencies of the forearm, the proximal radius at the elbow can be unstable and may subluxate anteriorly during extension. In a child with a congenital elbow disarticulation or transhumeral deficiency, an active elbow joint does not exist; hence, the child lacks the ability to grasp objects in the cubital fold. As the deficiency becomes increasingly proximal, as with shoulder disarticulations, it becomes increasingly difficult to perform functional activities. If the child has bilateral upper limb deficiencies at the more proximal levels, the child can work with occupational therapists to perform activities of daily living with their feet.[12]

Longitudinal deficiencies are not as common as transverse deficiencies. However, cases of radial longitudinal deficiencies have been associated with more complex medical syndromes. Radial longitudinal deficiency (RLD) is a congenital anomaly that presents with a deficiency along the radial side of the limb. It is 3 times as common as ulnar longitudinal deficiencies. It has varying degrees of involvement from thumb hypoplasia with an intact radius to the complete absence of the radius. It may occur bilaterally. Most cases of RDL result from spontaneous mutations; however, there are cases in which it may be autosomal recessive or dominant. Approximately one-third of RLD cases are associated with a syndrome that may involve the hematologic, cardiac, or renal systems. Radial longitudinal deficiency can be seen

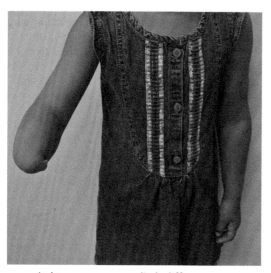

Fig. 1. Child with congenital transverse upper limb difference.

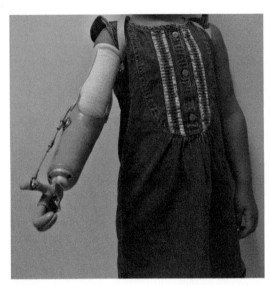

Fig. 2. Child with congenital transverse upper limb difference with body-powered prosthetic. (Prosthesis fabricated by SCOPe Orthotics and Prosthetics.)

in thrombocytopenia-absent radius syndrome, VACTERL (vertebral defects, anal atresia, cardiac malformation, tracheoesophageal fistula, esophageal atresia, renal anomalies, and limb anomalies) syndrome, Holt-Oram syndrome (cardiac septal defects), or Fanconi anemia. In those with less severe forms of RLD, such as thumb hypoplasia, treatment options may include opponensplasty, ulnar collateral ligament reconstruction, or pollicization depending on the level of involvement. For those with more severe forms of RLD, such as hypoplasia or absence of the radius, the shortened forearm may have a wrist that is radially deviated because of lack of bony support. This can lead to poor finger flexion and extension as the finger flexors and extensors are at a mechanical disadvantage. Surgical options, along with stretching and splinting, aim to maintain wrist and digit motion while centralizing the wrist relative to the forearm. The ultimate goal is to have a functional upper limb with a stable wrist and a functional oppositional thumb for pinch and grasp.[10,13]

Ulnar longitudinal deficiency is less common than RLD and often occurs in isolation and unilaterally. The entire limb can be hypoplastic and have abnormalities of the elbow and forearm. The hand and wrist are almost always affected. Up to 90% of patients may have missing digits.[10,11,14] As with RLD, the goal is to have a functional upper limb with an oppositional thumb and fingers.

Children with central upper limb deficiency, ectrodactyly, or cleft hand, sometimes referred to as lobster claw, have variable absence of the index, middle, and ring rays and central carpus. It can be inherited in an autosomal dominant pattern or occur spontaneously.[10] Longitudinal deficiency of the humerus is often associated with anomalies in the radius and ulna with phocomelic digits.[12]

When seeing a child with an upper limb difference, a history, including prenatal exposures and birth/family/developmental history and a thorough physical examination should be performed. A diagnostic workup, especially in a child with a radial longitudinal deficiency, should include:

- Echocardiogram
- Renal ultrasound scan

- Blood cell count
- Peripheral blood smear
- Spine radiographs
- Chromosomal challenge test, if Fanconi anemia is suspected

Lower Limb

Congenital lower limb differences occur less frequently than in the upper limb. The Centers for Disease Control and Prevention estimates that there are approximately 2 per 10,000 live births each year in the United States affected with congenital lower limb deficiencies.[1] Of these, the most common deficiencies are longitudinal toe reductions, longitudinal femoral deficiencies (proximal focal femoral deficiency [PFFD]), longitudinal fibular deficiencies, and longitudinal tibial deficiencies, in decreasing order.

Lower limb congenital malformations may progress with growth, depending on the extent and number of bones and growth plates involved. For example, in children with longitudinal fibular deficiency, the lateral femoral growth plate is often affected, causing progressive genu valgum. Most lower limb deficiencies are not associated with other organ system defects. Some exceptions are listed in **Table 1**.

In those with congenital lower limb differences, a comprehensive history and physical examination should be performed, including:

- Prenatal exposures and birth history
- Family history
- Developmental history, including gross and fine motor milestones
- Full review of systems to rule out possible syndromes, in particular, cardiac, musculoskeletal, eyes/ears/nose/throat, neurologic, gastrointestinal, and genitourinary
- Skin examination for dimples, scars, verrucous hyperplasia, breakdown, or other abnormalities; lymphedema associated with amniotic banding
- Joint assessment to determine stability and weight-bearing potential. Measure active and passive joint range of motion. Specifically, hip or knee dislocation and ankle stability are very important factors in surgical planning. Voluntary movement of the joint is also helpful in determining the child's ability to use it in combination with a prosthesis or orthosis in the future. If the child is able to cooperate, perform quantitative strength testing.
- Spine examination for scoliosis or overlying skin abnormalities

Table 1
Lower limb deficiencies associated with other organ system defects

Lower Limb Deficiency	Associated Organ System Defects[7,9,12]
Tibial deficiency	Deafness, ectrodactyly or polydactyly of the hands, craniofacial abnormalities
Femoral hypoplasia-unusual facies syndrome	Bilateral femoral deficiency, facial abnormalities including micrognathia and cleft palate, hypoplasia or synostosis of the upper extremity, vertebral abnormalities, congenital heart disease, and polydactyly
Roberts or SC phocomelia syndrome	Bilateral symmetric tetraphocomelia, thumb aplasia, syndactyly, elbow and knee flexion contractures, mental retardation, cleft lip/palate, micrognathia, hypotelorism, cryptorchidism, and cardiac defects
Sacral agenesis	Hemipelvectomy or hip disarticulation, and is often associated with neurogenic bowel and bladder

- Observation to determine if the child has sufficient seated/standing balance
- Assessment of achieved mobility (eg, commando, bear, or reciprocal crawling). Note if the child attempts to pull to stand on objects in the room. Observe ambulation, if present.
- Sensory testing, if able
- A full physical examination to rule out major organ abnormalities (such as cardiac defects)
- Labs/Imaging
  - If syndromic findings present on examination, consider appropriate genetic testing or consultation.
  - Radiographs of the involved limb with opposite side comparison can be helpful in determining outcomes and possible surgical planning. A scanogram can help determine total limb length discrepancy at maturity in the child that can stand in combination with bone age. Consider spine films if abnormalities are observed on examination. It is important to remember that in the newborn, radiographs are often not conclusive because of the lack of bony ossification.
- Formal gait analysis should be considered for abnormal gait patterns, difficulty with functional prosthetic fitting, or surgical planning, when available.[15]

Other Limb Differences

In addition to the transverse and longitudinal limb differences mentioned earlier, there are myriad musculoskeletal and neuromuscular conditions that affect the limbs—congenital radioulnar synostosis, talipes equinovarus (club foot), and leg length discrepancy, to name a few.

Arthrogryposis and arthrogryposis multiplex congenita are terms used to describe infants or children who have multiple congenital contractures. Arthrogryposis implies that the contractures affect multiple body areas (ie, more than just club feet.) There are more than 400 conditions described as having multiple congenital joint contractures. The most common type of arthrogryposis is amyoplasia. Amyoplasia is a condition in which the newborn lacks muscular development and growth with multiple joint contractures. In these cases, the skeletal muscle is replaced by dense fibrous tissue and fat. Arthrogryposis is associated with fetal akinesia (decreased fetal movement.) In addition to the multiple joint contractures, they may also have osteoporosis caused by decreased fetal limb movement. The condition is usually nonprogressive and may improve over time with physical therapy and splinting, but surgical intervention is often necessary.[16,17]

ACQUIRED AMPUTATIONS

In the pediatric population, acquired amputations most commonly occur from trauma and disease (ie, neoplasm, infections), with trauma being twice as common as disease. Traumatic amputations can result in permanent physical damage and disability and psychological trauma and affect future functionality or goals. Most traumatic amputations occur in men.

In a retrospective study done over a 12-year period in the United States, more than 91% of the traumatic amputations were finger amputations, especially in the age group 0 to 2 years, with doors being involved in most cases. Adolescent males experience a higher proportion of more serious amputation injuries.[6] Greater than 90% have single limb involvement. Of the more serious amputation injuries, 60% affect the lower limb. Lawn mower accidents, bicycle chains or spokes, tools, and motor vehicle collisions also contribute to pediatric amputations.

Aside from the physical, emotional, and psychological effects a traumatic amputation can have on a child and their family, the financial cost can also be a stressor. Acute care costs in train injuries resulting in amputation averaged more than $50,000 in one study, most of which involved the lower limb and usually required multiple debridements and revisions.[18] In another study, over a 10-year period, the average cost was $22,000, and most of these injuries were caused by power lawn mowers. Lawn mower injuries cause 11.1 injuries per 100,000 US children per year.[19] Of those, almost half are caused by the power lawn mower being operated in reverse. Prosthetic costs from time of injury to age 18 years can range from $73,000 to $116,000 per single lower limb amputation. With an average of 600 pediatric amputations every year from lawn mower injuries, the annual burden of cost ranges from $44 to $75 million.[20] Gunshot wounds caused the longest length of stay, highest number of procedures, and highest cost.[21] Fireworks are also a common cause of traumatic amputations, usually affecting the upper limb, with an average patient age of 9 years.[22] Farm equipment is a common cause of traumatic amputation in rural areas. It is estimated that in the United States, 200 children per year have orthopedic injuries severe enough for hospitalization from farm equipment. Younger children are more likely to be injured from falling off equipment or being run over, whereas older children become injured while riding or operating it.[23]

- Rural areas: farm injuries, lawn mower injuries, high-tension wire injuries
- Younger children: doors, lawn mowers, tools, household injuries
- Older children: lawn mowers, power tools, bicycles, fireworks, burns, gunshot wounds

Education, safety, and prevention (ie, door stop being placed above child's reach) can help prevent traumatic amputations.

Diseases and their complications can lead to amputations. Neoplasms are a frequent cause of disease-related limb amputations.

- Some tumor types that may result in amputation: osteogenic sarcoma, Ewing's sarcoma, rhabdomyosarcoma
- Highest incidence: ages 12 to 21 years
- Limb salvage versus amputation depends on
  - Aggressiveness of tumor
  - Stage
  - Responsiveness to neoadjunct therapy
  - Likelihood of getting tumor-free margins
- Thanks to advances in treatment, survival rates have gone from 15% in the 1970s to 60%–70% with surgery and chemotherapy.

In the event of limb salvage procedures, if a child has an endoprosthesis, they cannot participate in any contact sports (usually met with variable compliance).[12] Several studies have shown equivalent survival rates and long-term outcomes of those having limb salvage procedures versus amputation, with the exception that children undergoing limb salvage have higher complication rates.[24] For intercalary injuries, including neoplasm, the Van Nes rotationplasty may offer superior results than high amputation. In this surgery, the distal limb (the part of the limb farthest away from the body's center) is attached to the proximal limb (the part of the limb closest to the body's center) with the foot facing backwards. The foot/ankle then acts like the knee joint and a prosthesis is attached to it. This allows the patient improved control of the prosthesis, including the ability to ascend or descend stairs and inclines.

Complications from infections can also lead to amputations. Purpura fulminans can be caused by meningococcal septicemia as well as staphylococcus and streptococcus infections. It is characterized by rapidly progressive hemorrhagic necrosis of the skin and thrombosis. Infectious emboli from meningococcal septicemia may cause autoamputation of the digits or limbs. In addition to the amputation, frequently in multiple limbs, growth plates may be affected leading to angular deformities of the limb during growth. Skin may also be affected, possibly requiring skin graphs and prolonged wound care management to maintain skin integrity.[12] The patient and physician may decide to fit one, some, or all amputated limbs with prostheses depending on the use, functional need, and preference.

COMPLICATIONS POSTAMPUTATION

After a major life event, such as an amputation, there needs to be physical, mental, emotional, and psychological healing.

Pain can occur immediately postoperatively, and phantom limb pain is unique to those with amputations. Phantom limb pain is a painful sensation perceived in the missing limb after an amputation. Phantom limb pain can occur in 40% to 85% of the adult population with amputations.[25] In the pediatric population, phantom limb pain can also occur but rarely occurs in children younger than 10 years.[12] In a sample of 25 pediatric patients who underwent amputations caused by tumors, 19 of 25 (76%) had phantom limb pain within that first year postoperatively. However, by 1 year, only 2 had phantom pain (3 patients died during that year, and the other patient was discharged from the institution.) Treatment options may include oral medications (gabapentin, tricyclics), perioperative epidural analgesia, or peripheral nerve blocks.[26] In one study, patients who underwent body scan exercises and mental/guided imagery had an overall decrease in phantom limb pain.[27] Although the study was small, mirror therapy also shows promise in managing phantom limb pain.[28]

Terminal bony overgrowth can occur in children with acquired amputations through a bone and in congenital limb deficiencies. The terminal overgrowth results from the development of appositional new bone on the end of the residual limb.[7] It can cause pain, bursitis, and, if left untreated, can penetrate the skin.

Other complications postamputation may include[29]:

- Pain from overuse syndromes from compensatory techniques, low back pain from altered gait, neuroma
- Joint contractures
- Heterotopic ossification
- Dermatologic and skin concerns, including wound dehiscence, skin breakdown/ulcers, verrucous hyperplasia, dermatitis, folliculitis, and hyperhidrosis
- Psychologically grieving limb loss, depression, body-image concerns, posttraumatic stress disorder
- Poor fit with prosthesis

CLINICAL MANAGEMENT

A multidisciplinary/interdisciplinary approach is recommended when available, with biannually coordinated assessments by the physician, physical therapist, occupational therapist, prosthetist, social worker, psychologist, and nurse. In addition to managing the medical complications, the physiatrist can assist with the patient's life care plan to include potential changes in function/functional goals, medical concerns that may be encountered as the patient ages, planning for a prosthesis, adaptive equipment, therapies, psychological needs, and peer support.[30] The physical therapist can assist with contracture prevention, core strengthening, balance, gait, endurance, and work on a home exercise program. The occupational therapist can evaluate activities of daily living and assist with adaptive fitting, and, in the case of concomitant upper limb involvement, the patient may need to learn how to use his or her feet for activities and will need to remove the prosthesis for foot use. The prosthetist inspects the integrity of the prosthesis and makes adjustments for growth as necessary to ensure adequate fit in collaboration with the physician. A social worker and psychologist are often needed to assess the patient and family for psychosocial risk factors, depression, problems with self-image/self-esteem, acceptance of disability, and bullying or other school issues. Multidisciplinary management best ensures holistic care of a developing, growing child with a limb difference or acquired amputation. In the community-based practice in which a multidisciplinary approach is unavailable, physician follow-up should be coordinated with the prosthetist whenever possible. Fitting a prosthesis should be considered along with the age and developmental milestones of the child with a congenital limb difference.

In children with an upper limb difference or acquired amputation, a review of the last 25 years of English-language publications has found that prosthesis use rejection is 45% with body-powered prosthetics and 35% rejection rates with myoelectric prosthetics (these rates are much higher than those in the adult population of 26% and 23%, respectively.)[31] For those that choose to use a prosthetic arm, there are many options for terminal devices which the pediatric patient may want to use for task-specific skills (**Figs. 3–5**).

The ability to bear weight and ambulate should be evaluated as early as possible in the child with lower limb difference or acquired amputation, and all appropriate surgical or prosthetic options should be presented to the family. Sometimes surgery is needed to make the limb amenable to prosthetic fitting and improve function, or limb salvage/lengthening procedure may be appropriate. Often, this discussion can be postponed until the child has met the gross motor milestone of pulling to stand. Parents may opt to wait for any surgical intervention until the child is old enough to make the decision, often necessitating the physician and prosthetist to use creative solutions for functional prosthetic fitting around a limb deformity.

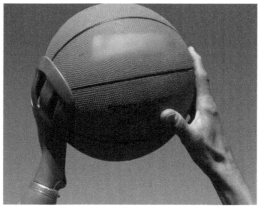

Fig. 3. Terminal device for basketball. (*Courtesy of* TRS Prosthetics, Boulder, CO; with permission.)

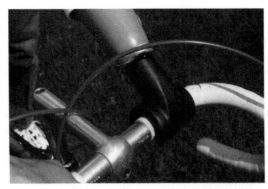

Fig. 4. Terminal device for cycling. (*Courtesy of* TRS Prosthetics, Boulder, CO; with permission.)

Initially, children may need a Silesian or waist belt for improved suspension, particularly if they are still transitioning from crawling or have bilateral limb deficiencies. Contrary to the adult amputee, intensive physical therapy for gait training is seldom needed, and gait aides often are only transitionally necessary and can sometimes be circumvented by the use of push-type toys in the young child.

For above-knee or knee-disarticulation amputees, the timing of the addition of a mechanical knee unit is still somewhat controversial. Usually, children are fit with a knee unit between ages 3 and 5 years, with concomitant physical therapy for gait training and safety. For bilateral lower limb involvement, fitting them with manual locking knees for comfort when sitting is often more appropriate because of risk of falls. These can be unlocked by the prosthetist one at a time for free-swinging use in gait when the child shows sufficient strength and balance.

The prosthesis should be reviewed by the prosthetist frequently and modified for growth, usually every 4 to 6 months. When growth velocity slows and limb volume is constant, adult-type of suspension systems may be introduced, such as suction or vacuum sockets.

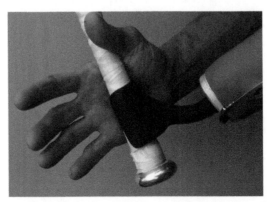

Fig. 5. Terminal device for holding a baseball bat. (*Courtesy of* TRS Prosthetics, Boulder, CO; with permission.)

Children often prefer to ambulate without their prosthesis at home, even after amputation. Home environment and equipment, such as arm crutches/walker and bath seat should be provided where appropriate.[7,9,10]

Presence of knee or ankle function can drastically improve options for surgical conversion and prosthetic fitting. For example, in the case of PFFD, the presence of ankle range of motion/stability with lack of knee function may offer possibilities of Van Nes rotationplasty surgery. This option offers superior control and function over a mechanical prosthetic knee (**Figs. 6** and **7**).

In devising a prescription for a child, the patient and family goals, aim for functionality, and aesthetic concerns must be taken into account. When selecting a prosthesis, one may compromise function for aesthetics and vice versa. Therefore, the clinician must identify the child's and family's priorities.[32] In children with upper limb prosthetic needs, there are options or opportunities for adults that are not yet available to younger patients, such as targeted muscle reinnervation, prostheses with combined motions with multiple degrees of movement, or multiarticulated prosthetic hands.

In patients with lower limb amputations, activity levels have generally been classified by the Medicare Functional Classification Level, or K-level. K-level is defined as a subjective assessment of current activity level of the amputee based on self-report and clinical observation (**Table 2**).

Children are often classified as K4 level. A proposed measurement of community-based gait performance in children is the quantified data collected by an ankle-worn accelerometer, worn over a particular time period.[33] However, this measurement has yet to be widely applied in pediatric amputees. Questionnaires such as the

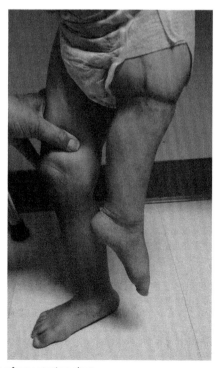

Fig. 6. Child with PFFD after rotationplasty.

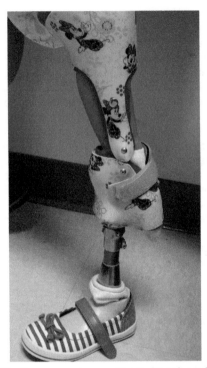

Fig. 7. Same child from **Fig. 6**, now wearing prosthesis. (Prosthesis fabricated by Loma Linda University Department of Prosthetics and Orthotics.)

Prosthetic Profile of the Amputee and Prosthesis Evaluation Questionnaire have not yet been validated in the pediatric population. This remains an area in need of further research. Subjective measures of prosthetic use/fit can include extracurricular activity, pain assessments, and skin evaluation.[15]

Table 2 K-levels		
K0	Functional Level 0	The patient does not have the ability or potential to ambulate or transfer safely with or without assistance, and a prosthesis does not enhance quality of life or mobility.
K1	Functional Level 1	The patient has the ability or potential to use a prosthesis for transfer or ambulation on level surfaces at fixed cadence. (Limited and unlimited household ambulator.)
K2	Functional Level 2	The patient has the ability or potential for ambulation with the ability to traverse low-level environmental barriers, such as curbs, stairs, or uneven surfaces. (Limited community ambulator.)
K3	Functional Level 3	The patient has the ability or potential for ambulation with variable cadence. Community ambulator who has the ability to navigate most environmental barriers.
K4	Functional Level 4	The patient has the ability or potential for prosthetic ambulation that exceeds basic ambulation skills, exhibiting high impact, stress, or energy levels. (Child, active adult, or athlete.)

SUMMARY

Congenital limb deficiencies are uncommon skeletal birth defects that may go undetected even with prenatal screening ultrasound scans. The most common etiology of acquired amputation is trauma. These children may have medical complications that prove challenging to manage. However, with a multidisciplinary/interdisciplinary team working with the child and family, the child can lead a successful, functional, and fulfilling life.

RESOURCES

- Association of Children's Prosthetic-Orthotic Clinics www.acpoc.org
- Amputee Coalition of America www.amputee-coalition.org
- US Paralympics www.usparalympics.org
- Challenged Athletes Foundation www.challengedathletes.org
- Disabled Sports USA www.dsusa.org
- Limbless Association www.limbless-association.org
- Limbs for Life Foundation www.limbsforlife.org
- National Amputee Golf Association www.nagagolf.org
- The Limb Connections www.LimbConnections.org
- Little Fins www.littlefins.org
- Limb Difference organization limbdifferences.org
- PFFD www.pffd.org
- Amputee-Online (www.amputee-online.com)

REFERENCES

1. Centers for Disease Control and Prevention. Available at: http://www.cdc.gov/ncbddd/birthdefects/ul-limbreductiondefects.html#ref. Accessed May 22, 2014.
2. Desrosiers TA, Herring AH, Shapira SK, et al. Paternal occupation and birth defects: findings from the National Birth Defects Prevention Study. Occup Environ Med 2012;69:534–43.
3. Werler MM, Pober BR, Nelson K, et al. Reporting accuracy among mothers of malformed and nonmalformed infants. Am J Epidemiol 1989;129:415–21.
4. McGuirk CK, Westgate MN, Holmes LB, et al. Limb deficiencies in newborn infants. Pediatrics 2001;108:e64.
5. Yoon PW, Rasmussen SA, Lynberg MC, et al. The national birth defects prevention study. Public Health Rep 2001;116(Suppl 1):32–40.
6. Hostetler SG, Schwartz L, Shields BJ, et al. Characteristics of pediatric traumatic amputations treated in hospital emergency departments: United States, 1990-2002. Pediatrics 2005;116:e667.
7. Smith DG, Michael JW, Bowker JH, et al. Atlas of amputations and limb deficiencies: surgical, prosthetic, and rehabilitation principles. 3rd edition. Rosemont (IL): American Academy of Orthopedic Surgeons; 2004. p. 773–914.
8. Bryant PR, Pandian G. Acquired limb deficiencies: 1. acquired limb deficiencies in children and young adults. Arch Phys Med Rehabil 2001;82(Suppl 1):S3–8.
9. Herring JA, Birch JG. The child with a limb deficiency. 1st edition. Rosemont (IL): American Academy of Orthopedic Surgeons; 1998.
10. Dy CJ, Swarup I, Daluiski A, et al. Embryology, diagnosis, and evaluation of congenital hand anomalies. Curr Rev Musculoskelet Med 2014;7:60–7.
11. Kozin SH. Upper extremity congenital anomalies. J Bone Joint Surg Am 2003;85-A:1564–76.

12. Alexander MA, Matthews DJ. Pediatric rehabilitation: principles and practice. 4th edition. 2010. p. 335–60.
13. Goldfarb CA, Wall L, Manske PR, et al. Radial longitudinal deficiency: the incidence of associated medical and musculoskeletal conditions. J Hand Surg 2006;31:1176–82.
14. Bednar MS, James MA, Light TR, et al. Congenital longitudinal deficiency. J Hand Surg 2009;34:1739–47.
15. Available at: http://now.aapmr.org/peds/musculoskeletal/Pages/Congenital-Lower-Limb-Deficiency.aspx. Accessed May 1, 2014.
16. Hall JG. Arthrogryposis (multiple congenital contractures): diagnostic approach to etiology, classification, genetics, and general principles. Eur J Med Genet 2014;57:464–72.
17. Bernstein RM. Arthrogryposis and Amyoplasia. J Am Acad Orthop Surg 2002; 10(6):417–24.
18. Blazer PE. Train injuries in children. J Orthop Trauma 1997;11(2):126–9.
19. Vollman D, Smith GA. Epidemiology of Lawn-Mower-related injuries to children in the United States, 1994-2004. Pediatrics 2006;188(2):e273–8.
20. Loder RT, Dikos GD, Taylor DA, et al. Long-term extremity prosthetic costs in children with traumatic lawnmower amputations. Arch Pediatr Adolesc Med 2004; 158:1177–81.
21. Trautwein LC, Smith DG, Rivara FP, et al. Pediatric amputation injuries: etiology, cost, and outcome. J Trauma 1996;41(5):831–8.
22. Moore RS, Tan V, Dormans JP, et al. Major pediatric hand trauma associated with fireworks. J Orthop Trauma 2000;14(6):426–8.
23. Lubicky JP, Feinberg JR. Fractures and amputations in children and adolescents requiring hospitalizations after farm equipment injuries. J Pediatr Orthop 2009;29: 435–8.
24. Nagarajan R, Neglia JP, Clohisy DR, et al. Review article: limb salvage and amputation in survivors of pediatric lower-extremity bone tumors. what are the long-term implications? J Clin Oncol 2002;20:4493–501.
25. Ehde DM, Czerniecki JM, Smith DG, et al. Chronic phantom sensations, phantom pain, residual limb pain, and other regional pain after lower limb amputation. Arch Phys Med Rehabil 2000;81(9):742–51.
26. Burgoyne LL, Billups CA, Jiron JL, et al. Phantom limb pain in young cancer-related amputees: recent experience at St. Jude Children's Research Hospital. Clin J Pain 2012;28(3):222–5.
27. McIver K, Lloyd DM, Kelly S, et al. Phantom limb pain, cortical reorganization, and the therapeutic effect of mental imagery. Brain 2008;131:2181–91.
28. Ramachandran VS, Rogers-Ramachandran D. Synaesthesia in phantom limbs induced with mirrors. Proc Biol Sci 1996;263:377–86.
29. Yoo S. Complications following an amputation. Phys Med Rehabil Clin N Am 2014;25:169–78.
30. Meier RH III, Choppa AJ, Johnson CB, et al. The person with amputation and their life care plan. Phys Med Rehabil Clin N Am 2013;24:467–89.
31. Biddiss EA, Chau TT. Upper limb prosthesis use and abandonment: a survey of the last 25 years. Prosthet Orthot Int 2007;31(3):236–57.
32. Passero T. Devising the prosthetic prescription and typical examples. Phys Med Rehabil Clin N Am 2014;25:117–32.
33. Pasquina PF, Bryant PR, Huang ME, et al. Advances in amputee care. Arch Phys Med Rehabil 2006;87:S34–43.

Pediatric Spinal Cord Injury
A Review by Organ System

Aaron Powell, MD[a],*, Loren Davidson, MD[b,c]

KEYWORDS

- Pediatric spinal cord injury • Spinal cord injury without radiographic abnormality
- Spasticity • Autonomic dysreflexia • Temperature regulation • Phrenic pacer
- Neurogenic bladder • Neurogenic bowel

KEY POINTS

- Congenital and acquired pediatric spinal cord injuries (SCI) pose unique management challenges because of the dynamic nature of cognitive and physical development in the growing child and the impact of the SCI on this complex process.
- Care for children and adolescents with SCI should be developmentally based, using appropriate strategies to facilitate adjustment and maximize independence across the spectrum of physical and emotional maturity levels.
- The goal of SCI rehabilitation for children and adolescents is to maximize function and independence and to prepare them for a successful transition to adulthood.
- Depending on age at injury, the acquisition of certain skills (eg, bowel and bladder continence) may not be rehabilitation, but rather habilitation, because they may have never achieved this skill previously.

 Video of tendon transfer surgery accompanies this article at http://www.pmr.theclinics.com/

INTRODUCTION

Congenital and acquired pediatric spinal cord injuries (SCI) pose unique management challenges because of the dynamic nature of cognitive and physical development in the growing child and the impact of the SCI on this complex process. In this

Disclosure: The authors have identified no professionals or financial affiliations for themselves or their spouse.
[a] Department of Physical Medicine and Rehabilitation, University of California Davis Medical Center, University of California Davis Health System, 4860 Y Street, Suite 3850, Sacramento, CA 95817, USA; [b] Department of Physical Medicine and Rehabilitation, University of California Davis Health System, 4860 Y Street, Suite 3850, Sacramento, CA 95817, USA; [c] Department of Physical Medicine and Rehabilitation, Shriners Hospitals for Children — Northern California, 2425 Stockton Boulevard, Sacramento, CA 95817, USA
* Corresponding author.
E-mail address: aaron.powell@ucdmc.ucdavis.edu

Phys Med Rehabil Clin N Am 26 (2015) 109–132
http://dx.doi.org/10.1016/j.pmr.2014.09.002
1047-9651/15/$ – see front matter © 2015 Elsevier Inc. All rights reserved.

review, an overview is provided of pediatric SCI rehabilitation management, highlighting how it differs from adult SCI management. Care for children and adolescents with SCI should be developmentally based, using appropriate strategies to facilitate adjustment and maximize independence across the spectrum of physical and emotional maturity levels. Emphasis should be placed on a family-centered approach to patient care, given the central role of parents and family in a child or adolescent's life.[1] Adolescents may not identify with the traditional pediatric model of care but are often not appropriate for an adult rehabilitation unit, which creates additional challenges when choosing the optimal therapeutic environment. Ideally, children and adolescents would receive care in a setting with age-appropriate peers having similar disabilities. However, the low incidence of pediatric SCI in the United States and the multitude of regional pediatric rehabilitation centers make the reality of a dedicated SCI unit for this population difficult to maintain and may require patients to receive care a great distance from their home and extended peer and community support network. The goal of SCI rehabilitation for children and adolescents is to maximize function and independence and to prepare them for a successful transition to adulthood. Depending on age at injury, the acquisition of certain skills (eg, bowel and bladder continence) may not be rehabilitation, but rather habilitation, because they may have never achieved this skill previously. For this reason, goal setting in therapy must be developmentally appropriate and may require a staged approach, whereby advanced level skills for a young child are deferred to a later date.

EPIDEMIOLOGY

A population-based database for SCI in the United States does not exist, and, thus, the epidemiology of pediatric and adult SCI has been extrapolated from the National SCI Statistical Center database and the Shriners Hospital SCI database. Using these data sets, the annual incidence of SCI in the United States is estimated to be between 25 and 59 new cases per million.[2] Assuming an average of 40 cases/million, this incidence means approximately 12,400 new SCI as estimated for the year 2010.[2] Of these new injuries, approximately 3% to 5% of the SCIs are in individuals younger than 15 years.[1,3] In adolescents, as in adults, males outnumber females by a ratio of 4:1. The preponderance of males over females with SCI decreases with earlier age at onset, and by 3 years of age, the number of females with SCI equals that of male.[4]

The neurologic level of injury and degree of completeness of the SCI varies with age. For example, infants and younger children with tetraplegia are more likely to have upper cervical injuries (C1-3) compared with adolescents (C4-8), because of a disproportionately large head and underdeveloped neck musculature.[4] The International Standards for Neurological Classification of SCI (ISCSCI) is the means by which the neurologic level of injury and degree of completeness is determined. In children, the reliability of the ISCSCI motor and sensory scores is good for children 5 years of age and older.[5] However, the anorectal examination, which is a frequent determinant of completeness of injury, is less reliable in younger children and therefore makes comparison between children and adults challenging.

The most common cause of SCI in children and adolescents is motor vehicle crashes, followed by violence and sports.[4] Unique causes of SCI in children include trauma resulting from lap belt injuries, child abuse, and birth injuries; and nontraumatic causes, such as instability of the upper cervical spine seen in Down syndrome, spinal stenosis seen in skeletal dysplasias, and inflammatory conditions, such as juvenile rheumatoid arthritis.[6,7] The unique causes and pathophysiology seen in pediatric SCI are not only a consequence of small stature but are related to unique characteristics of the developing musculoskeletal system, which is exemplified by the phenomenon of SCI without radiographic abnormality (SCIWORA). In SCIWORA SCI, plain radiographs, computed tomography myelography, and dynamic flexion/extension studies are all normal, whereas MRI abnormalities are seen in approximately two-thirds of patients.[8] Inherent elasticity of the spine in children allows transient self-reducing intersegmental displacement of the vertebral column in response to external forces and is believed to be the pathophysiologic mechanism underlying SCIWORA.[9] Hyperelasticity of ligaments and joint capsules also contributes to risk of SCI in neonates during difficult labor and delivery, as shown by a cadaveric study by Leventhal.[10] The neonatal vertebral column was tolerant of stretch up to 5 cm (2 in) without disruption, but the spinal cord could withstand only 0.64 cm (0.25 in) of distraction without tearing. The incidence of SCIWORA decreases with advancing age and reduced elasticity of the vertebral column, with 64% of children age 5 years or younger at injury having SCIWORA compared with 19% to 32% of older children up to age 21 years.[1]

REVIEW BY SYSTEM
Neurologic

Spasticity
Spasticity is a component of the upper motor neuron (UMN) syndrome characterized by velocity-dependent resistance to passive range of motion resulting from an increase in tonic stretch reflexes and accompanied by exaggerated tendon jerks.[11] Spasticity is not immediately apparent after complete SCI during the period of spinal shock. Spinal shock is a temporary loss of spinal reflex activity occurring below the zone of injury and is associated with flaccid paralysis and absent muscle stretch reflexes.[12] The duration of spinal shock is variable but usually resolves within weeks of injury. Spasticity generally follows spinal shock but may be delayed for up to 2 months or more in some circumstances. SCI characterized by concomitant damage to the anterior horn cell, nerve root, or distal LMN (including cauda equina) are characterized by flaccid paralysis and may mitigate the development of spasticity.

Clinical assessment begins with a comprehensive clinical evaluation by an experienced interprofessional team: the foundation for treatment planning and decision making. Spasticity is not always undesirable, and the rehabilitation approach to its treatment must consider both the positive and negative effects. The art of spasticity management is determining what degree of spasticity may be tolerable and of functional benefit versus counterproductive and potentially injurious.

The management of spasticity must be individually tailored to achieve specific goals set forth and agreed on by both the patient and clinician team. Taking an incremental approach with a treatment hierarchy has traditionally been recommended.[13] For example, after excluding potential nociceptive factors exacerbating spasticity, physical therapy and modalities are introduced before consideration of oral medications or injections. If less invasive options are insufficient, more invasive orthopedic and neurosurgical treatments, such as tendon lengthening surgery or intrathecal baclofen pump implantation, would be considered.

Therapy plays a critical role in management of spasticity. Interventions used often include range of motion, prolonged passive muscle stretching via splinting, and education in a home program.[14] Evidence for long-term efficacy of passive physical treatments such as stretching is lacking,[14,15] although regular standing on a tilt table or standing frame is frequently encouraged to stretch hip, knee, and ankle flexors. Passive stretching may be more effective when combined with other modalities, such as application of heat,[16] cooling,[17] neuromuscular electrical stimulation,[14] or selective nerve blocks.[18] Functional electrical stimulation (FES) using a cycle has also been shown to reduce spasticity and preserve range of motion. In addition, hydrotherapy has been shown to help reduce spasticity and the amount of antispasmodic medication needed.[19]

Oral medications used for systemic treatment of generalized spasticity commonly include baclofen, diazepam, dantrolene sodium, tizanidine, and clonidine (**Table 1**). These medications differ in their mechanism of action, and little is known about the pharmacokinetics/dynamics in children. The choice of which medication to use is often based on clinical experience, commencing at a low dose, with careful titration to optimal dose,[20] and monitoring for adverse effects or detrimental changes in function, such as increased muscle weakness. Medications may be used in combination to achieve complementary or synergistic effects. Baclofen is usually the first choice,[21] with diazepam often added as an adjunct to baclofen, initially at night to assist with sleep and reduce nighttime spasms.[22] Clonidine or tizanidine may also be useful adjuncts to baclofen and are also initiated as a single nighttime dose, because of sedative side effects. Dantrolene may be preferred in spasticity related to supraspinal injury, such as traumatic brain injury, to avoid sedation caused by baclofen and diazepam, although concerns about liver toxicity limit its use and necessitate monitoring of hepatic function.[20,23]

Focal hypertonicity can be managed with intramuscular botulinum toxin (BTX) injections and phenol/alcohol neurolysis. Injections are most effective in children with dynamic muscle shortening caused by spasticity or dystonia that is localized to specific muscles and in children without significant contracture.[24] Children undergoing injection with BTX may require sedation for comfort if multiple muscles are injected. In contrast, neurolysis with phenol is a more technically difficult procedure, requiring precision to avoid sclerosis of surrounding structures, and is more likely to require sedation. Electrical stimulation or ultrasonographic guidance may be used for muscle localization when injecting BTX in muscles that are not easily palpated, whereas phenol requires a targeting method for injections to avoid iatrogenic injury.

BTX blocks signal transmission at the neuromuscular junction by preventing the release of acetylcholine from the presynaptic axon of the motor end plate.[25] BTX has been shown to be effective in adults with SCI; however, there are no randomized studies or studies in children with SCI. BTX use in small muscles may be an important adjunctive therapy to increase the therapeutic effect of antispasticity medications and intrathecal baclofen, resulting in a more focal effect, thereby improving the use of orthoses and the effectiveness of rehabilitation programs in patients with SCI.[26]

Dosing and dilution guidelines in children have not been established, but consensus statements, systematic reviews, and randomized controlled trials provide recommendations.[24,27] Considerations used in dosing include the child's weight, muscle size, location of muscle, and degree of spasticity. The period of clinically useful relaxation is typically 12 to 16 weeks, and it is recommended that injections be spaced at a minimum of 3-month intervals because of concern for neutralizing antibody formation.[24] Adverse events related to BTX are rare and include injection-site pain and focal muscle weakness.[24,28] Since 2009, the US Food and Drug Administration has required black box labeling on BTX products, cautioning that the effects of the BTX may spread from the area of injection to other areas of the body, causing symptoms similar to those of botulism. Coadministration of BTX and aminoglycosides or other agents interfering with neuromuscular transmission is contraindicated. Further research on use of BTX in children with SCI is needed to determine efficacy, dosing, and functional outcomes in this population.

Phenol perineural injections (or motor point blocks) have been used for several decades to reduce focal spasticity in patients with SCI.[29] The low cost of phenol is a significant advantage over BTX, but the need for electrical stimulation guidance and general anesthesia in children may offset any cost savings (**Fig. 1**). Duration of clinical effect varies between 3 and 18 months.[18,30] Phenol neurolysis is typically used for large proximal muscles, such as the biceps brachii, hip adductors, and hamstrings, but can also be performed in the posterior tibialis and gastrocnemius muscles, with minimal risk of sensory dysesthesia. Phenol injections have been combined safely with BTXs in children, and this combination allows an increased number of injections at the maximal recommended dose during 1 procedure.[31,32] Phenol has been shown to be safe in children, but transient sensory dysesthesias occur rarely and were reported at 0.4% in 1 study.[31,32]

Surgical management should be considered when spasticity causes significant functional impairments that are refractory to more conservative management. Most research on pediatric surgical spasticity management involves children with cerebral palsy. These procedures are also effective and widely used in spasticity of spinal origin.[33]

Intrathecal baclofen (ITB) therapy is highly effective in treating generalized spasticity in both children and adults. ITB is delivered to the intrathecal space via a catheter connected to an implanted pump in the abdomen. This method of delivery infers an advantage over oral baclofen, in that central nervous system depressive effects are minimized and dosages can be titrated to functional effect. A thorough patient assessment and careful selection are crucial for a successful outcome. Goals of treatment (whether they are to improve function, comfort, or care) need to be firmly established.[34] Patient and family education and close follow-up are essential. Cost and maintenance can be prohibitive for some families. The battery life of the newer pumps is approximately 7 years. A screening lumbar intrathecal bolus dose of baclofen is recommended to evaluate responsiveness and impact on abilities, as well as adverse effects, but these trials are not performed universally.[34,35] Catheter tips are typically positioned at C5-T2 in patients with spastic tetraplegia and T10-T12 in those with paraplegia. Both the 20-mL and 40-mL pumps measure 8.75 cm in diameter, but the 20-mL pump is 19.5 mm thick, whereas the 40-mL version is 26 mm thick. Depending on the reservoir size and the patient's dosing regimen, the refill interval is usually between 2 and 6 months. The surgical technique of placing pumps subfascially (see **Fig. 1**) as opposed to subcutaneously (**Fig. 2**) in children may result in better aesthetics and lower incidence of wound erosion.

Potential complications of ITB include infections, respiratory depression, cerebrospinal fluid (CSF) leaks, and catheter problems, such as disconnection, migration, or kinking. Pump malfunction is less common. In 1 study,[36] the most common complications of surgery were catheter-related problems (31%), seromas (24%), and CSFs (15%). ITB has not been found to significantly affect the rate of progression of scoliosis in children with cerebral palsy,[37,38] but no such studies exist in children with SCI. ITB withdrawal is a medical emergency and needs to be identified early and managed aggressively. Caregivers should have a home supply of oral baclofen and be instructed to administer it at first signs of baclofen withdrawal. Causes can

Table 1
Dosing guidelines, pharmacologic actions, and side effect profile of commonly prescribed oral antispasmodic medications for children

Oral Medication (Dose/Frequency, Age/Weight Range)	Mode of Action	Side Effects/Precautions
Baclofen (0.125–1 mg/kg/d) Dosing guideline 2–7 y: 2.5–10 mg 4 times a day (10–40 mg/d) 8–12 y: 5 mg 3 times a day to 15 mg 4 times a day (15–60 mg/d) 12–16 y: 5–20 mg 4 times a day (20–80 mg/d) Note: adult doses may reach up to 150–200 mg/d. Caution advised with renal impairment, consider reducing dose	Centrally acting, structural analogue of GABA, binds to $GABA_B$ receptors of presynaptic excitatory interneurons (and postsynaptic primary afferents), causing presynaptic inhibition of monosynaptic/polysynaptic spinal reflexes Rapid absorption, blood level peaks in 1 h, half-life 3–4 h Renal and hepatic (15%) excretion	CNS depression (sedation, drowsiness, fatigue), nausea, headache, dizziness, confusion, euphoria, hallucinations, hypotonia, ataxia, paresthesia Note: abrupt withdrawal may cause seizures, hallucinations, rebound muscle spasms and hyperpyrexia
Diazepam (0.12–0.8 mg/kg/d) Dosing guideline: 0.5–10 mg 3 times a day Note: prescription of a nighttime dose only or proportionately larger dose at bedtime may help to limit problems caused by sedation	Centrally acting, binds to $GABA_A$ receptors mediating presynaptic inhibition in brain stem reticular formation and spinal polysynaptic pathways Rapid absorption, blood level peaks in 1 h, with half-life of 20–80 h Metabolized in liver, producing pharmacologically active metabolites with long duration of action. Increased potential for side effects with low albumin levels because of being 98% protein bound	CNS depression (sedation, impaired memory and attention), ataxia Dependence/potential for substance abuse/ overdose Withdrawal syndrome (including anxiety, agitation, irritability, tremor, muscle twitching, nausea, insomnia, seizures, hyperpyrexia)
Dantrolene sodium (3–12 mg/kg/d) Dosing guideline (for children >5 y old) Commence at 0.5 mg/kg twice a day for 7 d, then 0.5 mg/kg 3 times a day for 7 d, then 1 mg/kg 3 times a day for 7 d, then 2 mg/kg 3 times a day to a maximum of 3 mg/kg 4 times a day or 400 mg/d[44,45]	Peripheral action, blocking release of calcium from sarcoplasmic reticulum with uncoupling of nerve excitation and skeletal muscle contraction Blood level peaks in 3–6 h (active metabolite 4–8 h), with half-life of approximately 15 h Metabolized largely in liver, with 15%–25% of nonmetabolized drug excreted in urine	Malaise, fatigue, nausea, vomiting, diarrhea, muscle weakness with high dose Note: hepatotoxicity (baseline liver function tests must be checked before starting dantrolene, tested weekly during dose titration and regularly every 1–2 mo thereafter). Drug should be discontinued promptly if liver enzyme levels become increased

Drug	Dosing guideline	Mechanism / pharmacokinetics	Side effects
Tizanidine	Dosing guideline: In children <10 y: commence 1 mg orally at bedtime initially, increasing to 0.3–0.5 mg/kg in 4 divided doses. In children >10 y: commence 2 mg orally at bedtime initially, increased according to response, maximum 24 mg/d in 3–4 divided doses[45]	Centrally acting, α_2-adrenoceptor agonist activity at both spinal and supraspinal sites. Prevents release of excitatory amino acids, facilitating presynaptic inhibition. Good oral absorption, blood level peaks in 1–2 h, with a half-life of 2.5 h. Extensive first-pass hepatic metabolism with urinary excretion of inactive metabolites	Dry mouth, drowsiness, tiredness, headache, dizziness, insomnia, anxiety, aggression, mood swings, visual hallucinations, risk of hypotension (although 10 times less antihypertensive potency than clonidine), nausea, vomiting and constipation[50]. Liver function tests should be monitored for increase in enzyme levels in view of possible hepatotoxicity
Clonidine	Dosing guideline 0.025–0.1 mg in 2–3 divided doses. Note: a retrospective chart review of literature about clonidine in children reported an average dosage based on weight was 0.02–0.03 mg/kg/d (0.4–0.5 mg/d), with a range of 0.0014–0.15 mg/kg/d[47]	Centrally acting, mixed α-adrenoceptor agonist with predominant α_2 activity causing membrane hyperpolarization at multiple sites in brain, brainstem, and dorsal horns of spinal cord. Inhibition of substance P may also contribute to tone reduction via an antinociceptive effect. Rapidly absorbed orally, blood level peaks in 1–1.5 h, with a half-life of 2.5 h	Drowsiness, dry mouth, bradycardia, orthostatic hypotension. Abrupt cessation may result in rebound hypertension

Abbreviations: CNS, central nervous system; GABA, γ-aminobutyric acid.

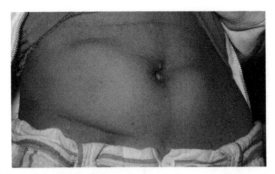

Fig. 1. A child with a subfascial baclofen pump.

include catheter problems, human programming error, failure to refill pump, or medication error.

Dysautonomia (autonomic dysreflexia and temperature regulation)

Lesions of the spinal cord at the T6 level and rostral result in autonomic nervous system dysfunction, manifesting as autonomic dysreflexia (AD) and impaired temperature regulation. The pathophysiology, symptoms, and criteria for diagnosis (systolic blood pressure increase of 20–40 mm Hg) of AD are the same in children and adults. More than half of children with T6 or higher injuries likely experience AD, with older children having typical symptoms, such as facial flushing, headaches, and piloerection; children younger than 5 years rarely show these signs and symptoms.[39] The key distinctions are that children have different normative blood pressures, and they may have more difficulty communicating the sometimes vague or abstract symptoms associated with AD.[39] Diligence in looking for signs of AD, timely intervention, and education in AD prevention for parents/caregivers and patients are tenets to avoiding the serious complications.

Impaired temperature regulation results from disruption of afferent input to thermoregulatory centers and impaired control of the distal sympathetic nervous system. As a result, persons with SCI are susceptible to a phenomenon known as poikilothermia, whereby the patient assumes the temperature of the outside environment, resulting

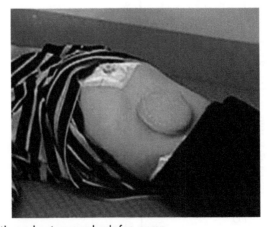

Fig. 2. A child with a subcutaneous baclofen pump.

in either hypothermia or hyperthermia.[40] Young children may be particularly suscep-tible to this complication, because of their inability to educate other caregivers, who may be less familiar with the risk of environmental exposure in SCI.

Respiratory

Respiratory complications from SCI are significant causes of morbidity and mortality in children.[41] Although a child with cervical level SCI may require initial ventilator support, many of these children are weaned from this support.[41] Children who are unable to be weaned require long-term ventilator support. This support can be provided by me-chanical ventilator or, in some cases, by a phrenic pacer (see **Fig. 2**), which stimulates either the phrenic nerve or the diaphragm muscle, directly resulting in muscular contraction and resultant inhalation. Exhalation with the phrenic pacer is dependent on passive recoil of the chest wall, and, thus, with increased need for secretion man-agement (such as in the setting of pneumonia) positive pressure ventilation is usually required. The advantages to phrenic pacing are that it is generally less invasive and mimics normal respiratory physiology more closely (**Fig. 3**).[42] Some children use a combination of both ventilation strategies.

Genitourinary

Neurogenic bladder

Similar to adults with SCI, the primary goals of neurogenic bladder management in children are to preserve renal function, prevent life-threatening complications, and promote continence.[43] Clinical Practice Guidelines from the Consortium of Spinal Cord Medicine[44] recommend use of clean intermittent urinary self-catheterization as the standard of care. Intermittent catheterization should be introduced at the age of 3 years, with the goal of obtaining complete independence by 5 to 7 years old, which mirrors the progression toward independent bladder management of the child's able-bodied peers. Children who do not have sufficient hand function to catheterize inde-pendently should gain independence in verbal direction of care. The importance of obtaining social continence in SCI is paramount, because of the social stigma associ-ated with foul odor and dependence on diapers, which may have devastating conse-quences for a child's social development, self-esteem, and societal integration.[45]

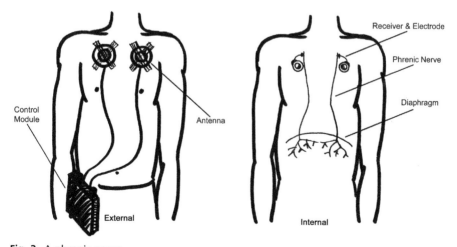

Fig. 3. A phrenic pacer.

The success of neurogenic bladder management in achieving continence is dependent on the ability of the bladder to store sufficient urine until self-catheterization can be performed. For children who do not obtain satisfactory continence with conservative methods, surgical intervention may be a consideration. With a spastic detrusor muscle, anticholinergic medications, detrusor BTX injections, or bladder augmentation may be required to increase bladder storage capacity.[46] Additional causes of incontinence may include an open bladder neck or weak urinary sphincter, resulting in stress incontinence. Incompetence of the bladder outlet may require urethral bulking injection agents, artificial urinary sphincter devices, or a bladder neck sling. In addition, in children with poor hand function, abductor strength, or females with difficulty mobilizing, a continent catheterizable urinary diversion (**Fig. 4**) has shown improved independence with catheterization, greater overall patient satisfaction, and few complications.[47–49]

Gastrointestinal

Neurogenic bowel

The goal of neurogenic bowel management in the child with SCI is achievement of continence in an expedient and practical manner, with prevention of complications.[43] Because neurogenic bowel function in adults with SCI is a similar physiologic process, many of the management principles are the same. Bowel programs can be successfully introduced around 2 to 4 years old.[50] There should be an attempt to distinguish between upper motor and lower motor neuron bowel (with the latter lacking bowel reflexes and peristalsis), because the management and bowel agents chosen may vary significantly. Although conservative measures such as use of the gastrocolic reflex, gravity-aided postures, and suprapubic pressure (Credé maneuver) should be trialed first, more than 80% of children require the use of either oral, rectal, or combination medication regimens (**Table 2**).[51]

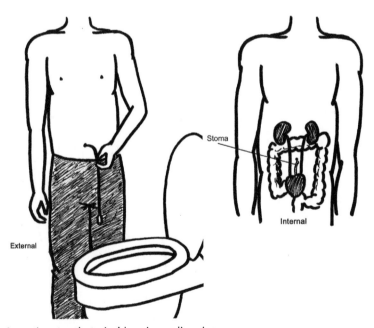

Fig. 4. A continent catheterizable urinary diversion.

Table 2
Dosing guidelines, pharmacologic actions, and side effect profile of commonly prescribed neurogenic bowel medications for children

Class	Medication (Dose/Frequency, Age/Weight Range)	Mode of Action	Side Effects/Precautions
Bulk forming	Psyllium (eg, Metamucil, Fibercon, Citrucel) Dosing guidelines <6 y: Safety and efficacy not established 6–12 y: 1.25–15 g/d orally in 227.3 mL (8 oz) of water in divided doses >12 y: 2.5–7.5 g in 227.3 mL (8 oz) of water orally, ≤30 g/d in divided doses	Absorbs water to create stool bulk	Bloating, flatulence, abdominal cramps, gastrointestinal obstruction, constipation
Stool softeners	Docusate (Colace, Surfak) Dosing guidelines Children 2–11 y: dose: 50–150 mg/d orally divided daily, twice a day ≥12 y: 50–300 mg/d orally divided daily, twice a day	Emulsifies stool fat and water, allowing mixture Metabolism is unknown	Diarrhea, abdominal cramps, rash, throat irritation, liquid form tastes bitter and is poorly tolerated
Hyperosmolar	Lactulose (1 mL/kg orally daily, twice a day) Dosing guidelines: maximum: 60 mL/d Note: response may require 24–48 h	Draw fluid into intestines increasing stool water content; it can also increase stool acidity, trapping NH4 ions Metabolized by colon; colon with <3% systemic absorption	Flatulence, intestinal cramps, abdominal distension, nausea, vomiting May cause electrolyte disorders or metabolic acidosis with excessive doses
	Sorbitol (25 g/120 mL,50 g/240 mL) Dosing guidelines: 1–12 y: 25–50 g orally once within 1 h of ingestion Note: not recommended for multiple dose treatment	Draws excessive water into the colon, promoting evacuation Not metabolized, because it is not absorbed systemically	Vomiting, constipation, black stools, diarrhea May cause electrolyte imbalance, fecal impaction, bronchiolitis obliterans
	Miralax (0.8 g/kg orally daily) Dosing guidelines: children <17 y: commence with 4 grams and progress to maximum of 17 grams fully dissolved in 113.6–227.3 mL (4–8 oz) of liquid before administration daily	Causes water retention in stool, producing laxative effect Not metabolized, because it is not absorbed systemically	Cramping, flatulence, nausea, abdominal distention, urticarial May cause electrolyte disturbance with prolonged and excessive use

(continued on next page)

Table 2
(continued)

Class	Medication (Dose/Frequency, Age/Weight Range)	Mode of Action	Side Effects/Precautions
Stimulants	Senna (Senokot) Dosing guidelines 2–5 y: 1 tab orally every night at bedtime as needed; start: half a tab every night at bedtime; maximum: 1 tab twice a day 6–11 y: 2 tabs orally every night at bedtime as needed; Start: 1 tab every night at bedtime; maximum: 2 tabs twice a day >12 y: 2–4 tabs orally every night at bedtime as needed; start: 2 tabs every night at bedtime; maximum: 4 tabs twice a day	Increases intestinal motility by stimulating peristalsis Liver metabolism, although minimal systemic uptake. Takes 6–12 h to work	Nausea, abdominal distension, cramps, flatulence, diarrhea, urine discoloration
	Bisacodyl (Dulcolax) Dosing guidelines 6–11 y: 1 tab orally daily as needed; do not cut/crush/chew >12 y: 1–3 tabs orally daily as needed; do not cut/crush/chew	Increases intestinal motility Metabolized by liver with 15% systemic absorption	Diarrhea, cramping, rectal sensation burning, vomiting, nausea
	Magnesium citrate Dosing guidelines 2–5 y: 2–4 mL/kg/d orally divided daily, twice a day; maximum: 60–90 mL/d 6–12 y: 100–150 mL/d orally divided daily, twice a day; maximum: 150 mL/d >12 y: 150–300 mL/d orally divided daily, twice a day; maximum: 300 mL/d	Stimulates colonic motility, used for complete bowel evacuation	Large volume, poor taste, electrolyte imbalance, hypotension, diarrhea, flatulence
	Milk of magnesia Dosing guidelines 6 mo–1 y: 40 mg/kg orally daily 2–5 y: 400–1200 mg orally daily 6–11 y: 1200–2400 mg orally daily >12 y: 2400–4800 mg orally daily	Neutralizes gastric acidity, which causes water retention in stool Not metabolized, with 15%–30% systemic absorption	Diarrhea, abdominal pain, nausea, dehydration, vomiting

	Drug / Dosing guidelines	Mechanism	Adverse effects
Enemas	Saline Dosing guidelines 2–12 y: 6 mL/kg (up to 118 mL) by rectum daily >12 y: 1 bottle (118 mL) by rectum daily	Hyperosmotic effect of sodium draws excess water into the colon, promoting evacuation Minimal systemic absorption	Abdominal distension, nausea, discomfort, electrolyte imbalance, metabolic acidosis Do not use in renal failure
	Mineral oil Dosing guidelines 2–11 y: 1/2 bottle by rectum daily >12 y: 1 bottle by rectum daily	Softens and lubricates stool Unknown metabolism with minimal systemic absorption	Diarrhea, abdominal cramps, pruritus
Suppositories	Bisacodyl (Dulcolax) Dosing guidelines 6–11 y: half a suppository by rectum daily >12 y: 1 suppository by rectum daily	Causes increased peristalsis by providing mild colonic irritation Liver metabolized, with 15% systemic absorption	Diarrhea, abdominal pain, nausea, dehydration, vomiting, electrolyte imbalance
	Glycerin Dosing guidelines <2 y: half infant/pediatric suppository by rectum daily 2–5 y: 1 infant/pediatric suppository by rectum daily >6 y: adult suppository by rectum daily	Irritates mucosa, increasing peristalsis; increases stool water content Liver metabolized with poor rectal absorption	Diarrhea, headache, nausea, rectal irritation

Additional strategies in children include the use of retrograde irrigation systems, such as cone enemas or inflatable rectal catheters (Peristeen system, Coloplast Ltd, UK).[52] Children with significant difficulty in achieving continence may benefit from an anterograde continence enema procedure, in which a stoma is made from the abdomen to the proximal colon (**Fig. 5**).[53] This procedure is well tolerated, has minimal side effects, and is generally effective in restoring continence.[54]

Endocrine: Hypercalcemia

Hypercalcemia is a serious complication, which can affect around 23% of children with SCI, particularly adolescent males.[55] The classic symptoms of hypercalcemia are abdominal pain, polyuria, vomiting, generalized malaise, and potential psychosis. A high index of suspicion should be maintained, because misdiagnosis may lead to unnecessary testing and treatment, including reported incidences of hypercalcemia leading to surgery for acute abdomen. Hypercalcemia is also associated with increased risk of nephrocalcinosis, urolithiasis, and renal failure.[55] Diagnostic evaluation should exclude alternative causes of increased serum calcium levels, such as parathyroid dysfunction or Paget disease. Treatment is generally aggressive hydration with furosemide diuresis, although bisphosphonates may be considered as well.[56]

Integument

Wounds in children with SCI are a devastating complication, because of the lack of protective sensation. Although wounds secondary to pressure phenomena are most common, burn injury is also seen in greater frequency. The true incidence of skin breakdown in children with SCI is not known; however, Shriners Hospitals for Children, Chicago[57] have reported around 21% prevalence in their pediatric SCI population, with up to 55% of children reporting pressuring ulcers within the first decade after injury. Risk factors for skin breakdown differ between children and adults with SCI.

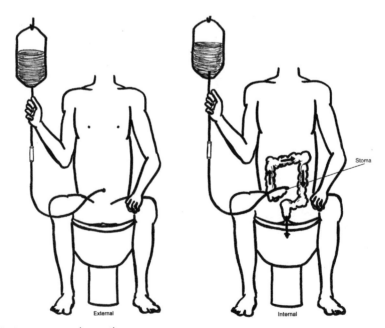

Fig. 5. An anterograde continence enema.

Although younger children may be prone to wounds because of their play, increased floor time, and limited cognitive understanding, body image issues and unwillingness to perform skin checks may increase risk in adolescents.[58] As the child matures, the physician must help facilitate incremental shifting of responsibility from the parents to the child in addition to reinforcing frequent pressure relief, appropriate fit of wheelchair and cushion, good hygiene, and proper nutrition.[1]

Vascular: Deep Venous Thrombosis

Deep venous thrombosis (DVT) is a rare complication in children with SCI.[59] The risk of DVT in children younger than 12 years is low enough that chemoprophylaxis is not routinely recommended, unless other significant risk factors are present.[60] Current clinical practice guidelines for DVT prophylaxis do not differentiate the indications for, or duration of, DVT prophylaxis in children versus adults. The treatment protocols for documented DVT are similar to those for adults, with the exception of weight-based dosing of low-molecular-weight heparin and the need for measurement of anti–factor Xa levels, because of variable rates of metabolism in children.[1]

Orthopedic

Scoliosis and hip dislocation/subluxation

Children with SCI are at unique risk for several orthopedic complications that do not occur in the skeletally mature adult. The first is scoliosis. Almost every child who sustains an SCI before skeletal maturity develops scoliosis, and approximately two-thirds of these children require surgery.[61] Thoracolumbar-sacral orthotic bracing has been shown to significantly slow the rate of curve progression and delay the need for surgery in children with SCI.[62] However, compliance with these often bulky and sometimes functionally limiting braces can be difficult.[63] Regardless, close surveillance and referral to surgery when appropriate are essential. General indications for spine fusion surgery in children with neurogenic scoliosis secondary to SCI include curves greater than 40° by Cobb angle, age greater than 10 years, rapid progression of the curve, and functional problems or pain in a mature patient.

The second most common orthopedic complication experienced by children with SCI is hip subluxation or dislocation. More than 90% of children with SCI before age 10 years develop hip subluxation or dislocation.[64] There is some evidence[65] that this complication occurs whether spasticity is present or not. Lack of hip joint integrity can inhibit the child's ability to use standing frames or FES bicycles, in addition to being a potential pain generator. Therefore, close surveillance of hips and an aggressive approach to surgical intervention are generally recommended.[66]

Like adults with SCI, children are also affected by heterotopic ossification (HO), osteopenia, and pathologic fractures. HO is less prevalent in children, although it still has an incidence around 3%.[67] It is also believed to show up later in children than in adults, occurring on average around 4 months after injury.[68] Children with SCI have been found to have 40% less bone density than age-matched and gender-matched controls.[69] This finding, in conjunction with increased activity and risk-taking behavior, may predispose to pathologic fracture. Close monitoring, education, and screening for treatable risk factors (eg, inadequate dietary intake of calcium and vitamin D) is warranted.

Upper extremity reconstruction

The most rapid neurologic recovery after SCI usually happens within the first 6 months to year after injury.[70] When the neurologic examination has stabilized, and further improvement in upper extremity function in the tetraplegic patient is not anticipated, surgical reconstruction of the upper extremity may be considered.[71] In the interim, rehabilitation management must focus on preservation of range of motion in the upper extremity using both active and passive stretch, orthoses, and spasticity management to avoid contracture development, which may preclude or complicate surgical options. Surgical reconstruction options may include tendon transfer, nerve transfer, implantation of an FES device, or a combination of these interventions. The goal of surgical intervention for the upper extremity in tetraplegic patients with SCI may be to restore function or simply balance the biomechanical forces about a joint to minimize the risk of progressive myostatic contracture. Realistic goal setting by patient and clinician before intervention are key to the perception of a successful outcome, because restoration of normal function is not possible. Of the available options, tendon transfer is the most commonly used and has the greatest amount of reported outcomes in the medical literature.

Neuroprosthesis/functional electrical stimulation FES of the upper extremity may be performed transcutaneously or via implanted electrodes. To be a candidate for FES, the target muscle must have an intact lower motor neuron (LMN) to be electrically excitable. It is common for both UMN-type and LMN-type injuries to be present with SCI, because the involvement of the anterior horn cell at the level of injury results in an LMN injury pattern, whereas the segments below this level show a UMN pattern. If the target muscle for a given action like wrist extension does not have an intact LMN, consideration can be given to transferring an alternative muscle donor amenable to electrical stimulation.[71]

Nerve transfer The restoration of function using nerve transfer involves sacrificing all or a portion of a donor nerve and its associated action to reinnervate and restore the function lost in the recipient nerve and target muscle.[72] The premise underlying nerve transfer is that the recipient nerve and muscle are of such functional importance that they supercede any loss associated with sacrificing the donor nerve.[73] Nerve transfer is rarely used, and most reports are limited to small case reports lacking long-term outcome, functional measures, or patient satisfaction.

Several fundamental principles have been reported to maximize outcome in motor nerve transfers[73,74]:

1. The recipient nerve should be repaired as close as possible to the target muscle to ensure the shortest amount of time for reinnervation and to minimize risk of distal nerve and motor endplate degeneration
2. Donor nerve should be from a muscle with function that is either expendable or that has redundant innervation
3. Nerve repair should be performed directly, without intervening graft
4. Use of a donor nerve with pure motor fibers maximizes muscle fiber reinnervation
5. Donor nerve should have many motor axons and be a reasonable size match to the recipient nerve
6. Using a donor nerve with synergistic function to the recipient facilitates cortical readaptation
7. Motor reeducation improves functional recovery postoperatively

The reported advantages of nerve transfer over tendon transfer include:

1. Longer immobilization period and a greater amount of intraoperative dissection with tendon transfer[72]
2. With nerve transfer, reconstruction of finger flexion and extension can be performed at the same setting[75]

3. The length-tension curve of the muscle-tendon unit is not disturbed with nerve transfer, because the origin and insertion of the tendon are not changed[72]
4. A single nerve transfer has the ability to reinnervate multiple muscle groups (eg, transfer of brachialis motor branch to anterior interosseous nerve restores thumb flexion [flexor pollicis longus (FPL)] as well as finger flexion [flexor digitorum profundus (FDP)])[72,73]
5. With partial nerve transfer, loss of donor nerve/muscle function is minimized through axonal sprouting of the remaining motor axon[76]

Tendon transfer The options for surgical restoration of function via tendon transfer are dependent on the available muscles that remain innervated. An algorithm proposed by Dr M. James (**Fig. 6**) provides a systematic approach to deciding which tendon

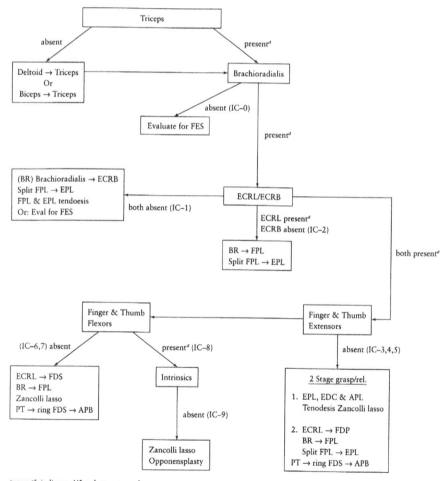

present[a]; indicates 4/5 or better strength.

Fig. 6. Algorithm for tendon transfer. APB, abductor pollicis brevis; APL, abductor pollicis longus; ECRB, extensor carpi radialis brevis (wrist extensor); ECRL, extensor carpi radialis longus; EPL, extensor pollicis longus; FDP, flexor digitorum profundus; FDS, flexor digitorum superficialis; FPL, flexor pollicis longus; IC, International classification; PT, pronator teres.

transfer may be indicated by motor examination of the upper extremity. The text that follows explains the reconstruction options with tendon transfer and the potential function that may be restored. Numerous variations of the described tendon transfer surgeries exist, and what follows is the approach in our institution as described by Dr M James. (Video 1)

Elbow extension

1. Surgery: deltoid to triceps or biceps to triceps tendon transfer
2. Function restored: elbow extension. May allow the patient to assist with transfers, perform pressure relief maneuvers, propel a wheelchair, and increase their reach and available work space

If the triceps muscle is paralyzed, it is recommended that elbow extension be reconstructed first. Postoperative immobilization of the elbow in extension is required and thus is not readily combined with other tendon transfers during the same surgical procedure. The deltoid to triceps transfer is more commonly used and preferred, because it does not significantly weaken shoulder abduction, even if the deltoid is partially paralyzed.[71] In comparison, the biceps to triceps transfer weakens elbow flexion; however, an intact brachialis muscle is usually sufficient to preserve elbow flexion against gravity.[75,77]

Key pinch (passive)

1. Surgery: brachioradialis (BR) to extensor carpi radialis brevis (wrist extensor) tendon transfer ± carpometacarpal arthrodesis or split FPL transfer
2. Function restored: tenodesis-driven key pinch allows the patient to hold a fork, toothbrush, pen, catheter, or other small object.

The presence of intact elbow flexion and extension, and an intact BR muscle, affords options for restoration of key pinch, even if all other muscles below the elbow are paralyzed.[71] Key pinch is established by transferring the BR to a wrist extensor and simultaneously tenodesing the extrinsic thumb flexor and extensor tendons to the radius. The restoration of wrist extension after this procedure allows for a tenodesis-driven key pinch, which is released by passive flexion of the wrist with relaxation. Additional procedures to stabilize the thumb may improve the competency of the key pinch and may be achieved via carpometacarpal or interphalangeal joint arthrodesis or transferring half of the FPL tendon to the extensor pollicis longus (EPL) tendon, which is referred to as a split FPL transfer.[71]

Key pinch (active)

1. Surgery: BR to FPL + tenodesis of EPL, split FPL transfer
2. Function restored: active (stronger) key pinch allows the patient to hold a fork, toothbrush, pen, catheter, or other small object

The presence of intact elbow flexion, extension and wrist extension (extensor carpi radialis longus [ECRL]) muscle allows for reconstruction of an active key pinch. In contrast to a tenodesis-driven key pinch, transfer of the BR to the FPL allows for active key pinch, which has the potential to be twice as strong, providing approximately 2 kg of pinch strength.[71] This procedure is typically coupled with tenodesis of the EPL to the radius and a split FPL transfer to stabilize the thumb.

Hook grasp

1. Surgery (2 phases)

Extensor phase: tenodesis of extrinsic finger extensors to the radius + hand intrinsic tenodesis

Flexor phase: BR is transferred to the FPL, and the ECRL is transferred to the FDP

2. Function restored: holding a cup and the ability to pull up trousers

The reconstruction of a hook grasp requires 2 active wrist extensors in addition to the BR and involves reconstruction of an active key pinch (as described earlier) and uses the remaining wrist extensor to power finger flexion. This transfer restores an active grasp (flexion) but does not provide active finger extension to release objects and therefore must be coupled with tenodesis of the extrinsic finger extensors to facilitate passive release of grasp. In addition, the lack of hand intrinsic function predisposes to metacarpophalangeal joint hyperextension, or clawing, which is addressed by hand intrinsic muscle tenodesis. This reconstruction is performed in 2 phases (described earlier), which are performed 3 months apart.

Opponensplasty

1. Surgery: pronator teres (PT) transfer to the ring finger; flexor digitorum superficialis (FDS), which can then be transfer to the abductor pollicis brevis
2. Function restored: adduction and opposition of the thumb to improve active key pinch

The opponensplasty serves to restore adduction and opposition of the thumb to improve active key pinch by counteracting the supination force of the FPL acting in the absence of thenar intrinsics.[78,79] This reconstructive option is appropriate for patients with intact PT and flexor carpi radialis (FCR) muscles. The FCR is not usually transferred, because it is the only active wrist flexor at this level and is of functional benefit. The opponensplasty is performed in conjunction with the active key pinch and staged grasp reconstruction, as described earlier.

Restoration of hand intrinsic muscle balance (Zancolli lasso)

1. Surgery: tenodesis of FDS tendons of digits 2-5 to the palmar surface of the A1 pulley
2. Function restored: prevents clawing of fingers with grasp

The Zancolli lasso is an intrinsic tenodesis procedure that tethers the FDS tendons of digits 2-5 to the palmar surface of the A1 pulley, resulting in dynamic metacarpophalangeal joint flexion when the wrist is extended.

Immunologic

Latex allergy

Approximately 6% to 18% of all children with SCI are allergic to latex,[80] and the pediatric SCI population is at an increased risk for development of this complication. Risk factors for development of allergy to latex include age at exposure (with younger ages being at higher risk) and number of repeated exposures. All efforts should be made to prevent exposure.

SUMMARY

Although it is a rare injury, the physiologic, psychosocial, and economic impact of SCI in the child is dramatic and far reaching. Despite this situation, many children with SCIs have shown inspirational resiliency and are able to lead meaningful and productive lives.[81,82] Preparing these children for success requires optimizing their health by recognizing and anticipating specific complications that are a result of SCI. It also necessitates a dynamic, developmentally appropriate rehabilitation program, which is family centered and adapts to the child's ever-changing physiology and ability. The potential for functional independence that results from a comprehensive rehabilitation program should be maximized for every level of SCI. Until a cure for SCI is available, neurorecovery and adaptive strategies will continue to fail to restore normal function in most cases. However, current research into the potential for restoration of function through either a biological cure for the injured spinal cord or the use of technology as a work-around to restore function using novel neural interfaces is increasing exponentially. Stem cell research continues to make strides in the daunting task of identifying potential treatments that will support the inherent self-restorative abilities of the human central nervous system.[83,84] Clinical trials in humans for stem cell–based or pharmaceutical-based therapies are few and generally exclude children, because of safety concerns. Simultaneously, the medical technology industry has virtually exploded with adaptive technology such as powered exoskeleton orthoses, brain machine interfaces, and limb reanimation through FES, epidural stimulation, and intraspinal microstimulation systems.[85] Although experimental devices and treatments with unclear safety profiles usually exclude children in the early stages, the pediatric rehabilitation community needs to ready itself for the possibility of clinical trials. To evaluate the efficacy of novel therapeutics in children with SCI, validated outcome measures appropriate for children are essential and should be a research priority.

SUPPLEMENTARY DATA

Supplementary data related to this article can be found online at http://dx.doi.org/10.1016/j.pmr.2014.09.002.

REFERENCES

1. Vogel LC, Betz RR, Mulcahey MJ. Spinal cord injuries in children and adolescents. Handb Clin Neurol 2012;109:131–48.
2. Devivo MJ. Epidemiology of traumatic spinal cord injury: trends and future implications. Spinal Cord 2012;50(5):365–72.
3. Kewalramani LS, Kraus JF, Sterling HM. Acute spinal-cord lesions in a pediatric population: epidemiological and clinical features. Paraplegia 1980;18(3):206–19.
4. DeVivo MJ, Vogel LC. Epidemiology of spinal cord injury in children and adolescents. J Spinal Cord Med 2004;27(Suppl 1):S4–10.
5. Mulcahey MJ, et al. The international standards for neurological classification of spinal cord injury: reliability of data when applied to children and youths. Spinal Cord 2007;45(6):452–9.
6. Achildi O, Betz RR, Grewal H. Lapbelt injuries and the seatbelt syndrome in pediatric spinal cord injury. J Spinal Cord Med 2007;30(Suppl 1):S21–4.
7. Wills BP, Dormans JP. Nontraumatic upper cervical spine instability in children. J Am Acad Orthop Surg 2006;14(4):233–45.
8. Grabb PA, Pang D. Magnetic resonance imaging in the evaluation of spinal cord injury without radiographic abnormality in children. Neurosurgery 1994;35(3):406–14 [discussion: 414].
9. Dachling Pang M. The child with a spinal cord injury. In: Betz RR, Mulcahey MJ, editors. Spinal Cord Injury Without Radiographic Abnormality (SCIWORA) in Children. 1st edition. American Academy of Orthopaedic Surgeons; 1996. p. 139–58.
10. Leventhal HR. Birth injuries of the spinal cord. J Pediatr 1960;56:447–53.
11. Sanger TD, Delgado MR, Gaebler-Spira D, et al. Classification and definition of disorders causing hypertonia in childhood. Pediatrics 2003;111(1):e89–97.

12. Kirshblum S, Campagnolo DI. Spinal cord medicine. In: Kirshblum SC, Denise I, editors. Spinal Cor Medicine. 2nd edition. New York: Lippincott Williams & Wilkins; 2011. p. 265–81.

13. Merritt JL. Management of spasticity in spinal cord injury. Mayo Clin Proc 1981; 56(10):614–22.

14. Hsieh JTC, Wolfe DL, Connolly S, et al., Spasticity After Spinal Cord Injury: An Evidence-Based Review of Current Interventions. Topics in Spinal Cord Injury Rehabilitation. 13(1). Summer 2007. p. 81–97.

15. Pin T, Dyke P, Chan M. The effectiveness of passive stretching in children with cerebral palsy. Dev Med Child Neurol 2006;48(10):855–62.

16. Lee GP, Ng GY. Effects of stretching and heat treatment on hamstring extensibility in children with severe mental retardation and hypertonia. Clin Rehabil 2008; 22(9):771–9.

17. Abd El-Maksouda G, Sharafb M, Rezz-Allahc S. Efficacy of cold therapy on spasticity and hand function in children with cerebral palsy. J Advanced Research 2011;2:319–25.

18. Kwon JY, Kim JS. Selective blocking of the anterior branch of the obturator nerve in children with cerebral palsy. Am J Phys Med Rehabil 2009;88(1):7–13.

19. Kesiktas N, Paker N, Erdogan N, et al. The use of hydrotherapy for the management of spasticity. Neurorehabil Neural Repair 2004;18(4):268–73.

20. Kopec K. Cerebral palsy: pharmacologic treatment of spasticity. US Pharm 2008; 33:22–6.

21. Tilton A, Vargus-Adams J, Delgado MR. Pharmacologic treatment of spasticity in children. Semin Pediatr Neurol 2010;17(4):261–7.

22. Mathew A, Mathew MC. Bedtime diazepam enhances well-being in children with spastic cerebral palsy. Pediatr Rehabil 2005;8(1):63–6.

23. Gracies JM, Nance P, Elovic E, et al. Traditional pharmacological treatments for spasticity. Part II: general and regional treatments. Muscle Nerve Suppl 1997;6: S92–120.

24. Graham HK, Aoki KR, Autti-Ramo I, et al. Recommendations for the use of botulinum toxin type A in the management of cerebral palsy. Gait Posture 2000;11(1): 67–79.

25. Koman LA, Mooney JF, Smith BP, et al. Botulinum toxin type a neuromuscular blockade in the treatment of equinus foot deformity in cerebral palsy: a multicenter, open-label clinical trial. Pediatrics 2001;108(5):1062–71.

26. Santamato A, Panza F, Ranieri M, et al. Effect of intrathecal baclofen, botulinum toxin type A and a rehabilitation programme on locomotor function after spinal cord injury: a case report. J Rehabil Med 2010;42(9):891–4.

27. Kawamura A, Campbell K, Lam-Damji S, et al. A randomized controlled trial comparing botulinum toxin A dosage in the upper extremity of children with spasticity. Dev Med Child Neurol 2007;49(5):331–7.

28. Delgado MR, Hirtz D, Aisen M, et al. Practice parameter: pharmacologic treatment of spasticity in children and adolescents with cerebral palsy (an evidence-based review): report of the Quality Standards Subcommittee of the American Academy of Neurology and the Practice Committee of the Child Neurology Society. Neurology 2010;74(4):336–43.

29. Gunduz S, Kaylon TA, Dursun H, et al. Peripheral nerve block with phenol to treat spasticity in spinal cord injured patients. Paraplegia 1992;30(11): 808–11.

30. Yadav SL, Singh U, Dureja GP, et al. Phenol block in the management of spastic cerebral palsy. Indian J Pediatr 1994;61(3):249–55.

31. Kolaski K, Ajizian SJ, Passmore L, et al. Safety profile of multilevel chemical denervation procedures using phenol or botulinum toxin or both in a pediatric population. Am J Phys Med Rehabil 2008;87(7):556–66.
32. Gooch JL, Patton CP. Combining botulinum toxin and phenol to manage spasticity in children. Arch Phys Med Rehabil 2004;85(7):1121–4.
33. Elbasiouny SM, Moroz D, Bakr MM, et al. Management of spasticity after spinal cord injury: current techniques and future directions. Neurorehabil Neural Repair 2010;24(1):23–33.
34. Albright AL. Intrathecal baclofen for childhood hypertonia. Childs Nerv Syst 2007; 23(9):971–9.
35. Dan B, Motta F, Vles JS, et al. Consensus on the appropriate use of intrathecal baclofen (ITB) therapy in paediatric spasticity. Eur J Paediatr Neurol 2010; 14(1):19–28.
36. Albright AL, Gilmartin R, Swift D, et al. Long-term intrathecal baclofen therapy for severe spasticity of cerebral origin. J Neurosurg 2003;98(2):291–5.
37. Shilt JS, Lai LP, Cabrera MN, et al. The impact of intrathecal baclofen on the natural history of scoliosis in cerebral palsy. J Pediatr Orthop 2008;28(6):684–7.
38. Senaran H, Holden C, Dabney KW, et al. The risk of progression of scoliosis in cerebral palsy patients after intrathecal baclofen therapy. Spine 2007;32(21): 2348–54.
39. Hickey KJ, Vogel LC, Willis KM, et al. Prevalence and etiology of autonomic dysreflexia in children with spinal cord injuries. J Spinal Cord Med 2004;27(Suppl 1): S54–60.
40. Petrofsky JS. Thermoregulatory stress during rest and exercise in heat in patients with a spinal cord injury. Eur J Appl Physiol Occup Physiol 1992;64(6):503–7.
41. Padman R, Alexander M, Thorogood C, et al. Respiratory management of pediatric patients with spinal cord injuries: retrospective review of the duPont experience. Neurorehabil Neural Repair 2003;17(1):32–6.
42. Onders RP, Elmo MJ, Ignagni AR. Diaphragm pacing stimulation system for tetraplegia in individuals injured during childhood or adolescence. J Spinal Cord Med 2007;30(Suppl 1):S25–9.
43. Merenda L, Brown JP. Bladder and bowel management for the child with spinal cord dysfunction. J Spinal Cord Med 2004;27(Suppl 1):S16–23.
44. Lapides J, Diokno AC, Silber SJ, et al. Clean, intermittent self-catheterization in the treatment of urinary tract disease. J Urol 1972;107(3):458–61.
45. McLaughlin JF, Murray M, Van Zandt K, et al. Clean intermittent catheterization. Dev Med Child Neurol 1996;38(5):446–54.
46. Akbar M, Abel R, Seyler TM, et al. Repeated botulinum-A toxin injections in the treatment of myelodysplastic children and patients with spinal cord injuries with neurogenic bladder dysfunction. BJU Int 2007;100(3):639–45.
47. Merenda LA, Duffy T, Betz RR, et al. Outcomes of urinary diversion in children with spinal cord injuries. J Spinal Cord Med 2007;30(Suppl 1):S41–7.
48. Mitrofanoff P. Trans-appendicular continent cystostomy in the management of the neurogenic bladder. Chir Pediatr 1980;21(4):297–305 [in French].
49. Chulamorkodt NN, Estrada CR, Chaviano AH. Continent urinary diversion: 10-year experience of Shriners Hospitals for Children in Chicago. J Spinal Cord Med 2004;27(Suppl 1):S84–7.
50. Gleeson RM. Bowel continence for the child with a neurogenic bowel. Rehabil Nurs 1990;15(6):319–21.
51. Goetz LL, Hurvitz EA, Nelson VS, et al. Bowel management in children and adolescents with spinal cord injury. J Spinal Cord Med 1998;21(4):335–41.

52. Del Popolo G, Mosiello G, Pilati C, et al. Treatment of neurogenic bowel dysfunction using transanal irrigation: a multicenter Italian study. Spinal Cord 2008;46(7): 517–22.
53. Malone PS, Ransley PG, Kiely EM. Preliminary report: the antegrade continence enema. Lancet 1990;336(8725):1217–8.
54. Herndon CD, Rink RC, Cain MP, et al. In situ Malone antegrade continence enema in 127 patients: a 6-year experience. J Urol 2004;172(4 Pt 2):1689–91.
55. Tori JA, Hill LL. Hypercalcemia in children with spinal cord injury. Arch Phys Med Rehabil 1978;59(10):443–6.
56. Lteif AN, Zimmerman D. Bisphosphonates for treatment of childhood hypercalcemia. Pediatrics 1998;102(4 Pt 1):990–3.
57. Kathryn JH, Caroline JA, Lawrence CV. Pressure ulcers in pediatric spinal cord injury. Topics Spinal Cord Injury Rehabilitation 2000;6(0):85–90.
58. Vogel LC, et al. Unique issues in pediatric spinal cord injury. Orthop Nurs 2004; 23(5):300–8 [quiz: 309–10].
59. Jones T, Ugalde V, Franks P, et al. Venous thromboembolism after spinal cord injury: incidence, time course, and associated risk factors in 16,240 adults and children. Arch Phys Med Rehabil 2005;86(12):2240–7.
60. Vogel LC, Anderson CJ. Spinal cord injuries in children and adolescents: a review. J Spinal Cord Med 2003;26(3):193–203.
61. Dearolf WW 3rd, Betz RR, Vogel LC, et al. Scoliosis in pediatric spinal cord-injured patients. J Pediatr Orthop 1990;10(2):214–8.
62. Mehta S, Betz RR, Mulcahey MJ, et al. Effect of bracing on paralytic scoliosis secondary to spinal cord injury. J Spinal Cord Med 2004;27(Suppl 1):S88–92.
63. Chafetz RS, Betz RR, Gaughan J, et al. Impact of prophylactic thoracolumbosacral orthosis bracing on functional activities and activities of daily living in the pediatric spinal cord injury population. J Spinal Cord Med 2007;30(Suppl 1):S178–83.
64. McCarthy JJ, Chavetz RS, Betz RR, et al. Incidence and degree of hip subluxation/dislocation in children with spinal cord injury. J Spinal Cord Med 2004; 27(Suppl 1):S80–3.
65. Rink P, Miller F. Hip instability in spinal cord injury patients. J Pediatr Orthop 1990; 10(5):583–7.
66. McCarthy JJ, Betz RR. Hip disorders in children who have spinal cord injury. Orthop Clin North Am 2006;37(2):197–202 vi-vii.
67. Garland DE. A clinical perspective on common forms of acquired heterotopic ossification. Clin Orthop Relat Res 1991;(263):13–29.
68. Garland DE, Shimoya ST, Lugo C, et al. Spinal cord insults and heterotopic ossification in the pediatric population. Clin Orthop Relat Res 1989;(245):303–10.
69. Moynahan M, Betz RR, Triolo RJ, et al. Characterization of the bone mineral density of children with spinal cord injury. J Spinal Cord Med 1996;19(4):249–54.
70. Ditunno JF Jr, Stover SL, Freed MM, et al. Motor recovery of the upper extremities in traumatic quadriplegia: a multicenter study. Arch Phys Med Rehabil 1992; 73(5):431–6.
71. Michelle A, James M. Chapman's orthopaedic surgery. 3rd edition. Philadelphia: Lippincott Williams & Wilkins; 2001.
72. Brown JM. Nerve transfers in tetraplegia I: background and technique. Surg Neurol Int 2011;2:121.
73. Senjaya F, Midha R. Nerve transfer strategies for spinal cord injury. World Neurosurg 2013;80(6):e319–26.
74. Midha R. Nerve transfers for severe brachial plexus injuries: a review. Neurosurg Focus 2004;16(5):E5.

75. Revol M, Cormerais A, Laffont I, et al. Tendon transfers as applied to tetraplegia. Hand Clin 2002;18(3):423–39.
76. Gordon T, Yang JF, Ayer K, et al. Recovery potential of muscle after partial denervation: a comparison between rats and humans. Brain Res Bull 1993;30(3–4): 477–82.
77. Friedenberg ZB. Transposition of the biceps brachii for triceps weakness. J Bone Joint Surg Am 1954;36A(3):656–8.
78. House JH. Reconstruction of the thumb in tetraplegia following spinal cord injury. Clin Orthop Relat Res 1985;(195):117–28.
79. Kelly CM, Freehafer AA, Peckham PH, et al. Postoperative results of opponensplasty and flexor tendon transfer in patients with spinal cord injuries. J Hand Surg Am 1985;10(6 Pt 1):890–4.
80. Vogel LC, Schrader T, Lubicky JP. Latex allergy in children and adolescents with spinal cord injuries. J Pediatr Orthop 1995;15(4):517–20.
81. Anderson CJ, Vogel LC. Employment outcomes of adults who sustained spinal cord injuries as children or adolescents. Arch Phys Med Rehabil 2002;83(6):791–801.
82. Nelson VS, Dixon PJ, Warschausky SA. Long-term outcome of children with high tetraplegia and ventilator dependence. J Spinal Cord Med 2004;27(Suppl 1): S93–7.
83. Dasari VR, Veeravalli KK, Dinh DH. Mesenchymal stem cells in the treatment of spinal cord injuries: a review. World J Stem Cells 2014;6(2):120–33.
84. Silva NA, Sousa N, Reis RL, et al. From basics to clinical: a comprehensive review on spinal cord injury. Prog Neurobiol 2014;114:25–57.
85. Lobel DA, Lee KH. Brain machine interface and limb reanimation technologies: restoring function after spinal cord injury through development of a bypass system. Mayo Clin Proc 2014;89(5):708–14.

Evaluation of Phrenic Nerve and Diaphragm Function with Peripheral Nerve Stimulation and M-Mode Ultrasonography in Potential Pediatric Phrenic Nerve or Diaphragm Pacing Candidates

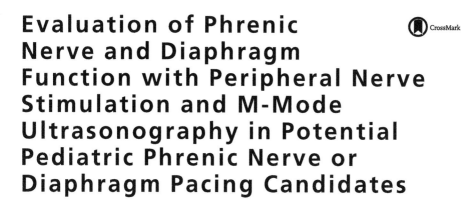

Andrew J. Skalsky, MD[a],*, Daniel J. Lesser, MD[b],
Craig M. McDonald, MD[c]

KEYWORDS

- Pediatric • Spinal cord injury • Diaphragm pacing • Phrenic nerve pacing
- Ultrasonography

KEY POINTS

- Combining phrenic nerve stimulation with observation of the movement of the hemidiaphragm with M-mode ultrasonography provides quantitative functional data in the setting of diaphragm paralysis.
- Traditional phrenic motor nerve conduction studies such as electromyography of the diaphragm have limitations in predicting the success of phrenic nerve or diaphragm pacing.
- Phrenic nerve pacing is an effective form of respiratory management in pediatric high cervical spinal cord injury.
- Successful phrenic nerve pacing in pediatric high cervical spinal cord injury can be accomplished with only one intact phrenic nerve and hemidiaphragm.
- Successful phrenic nerve pacing in pediatric high cervical spinal cord injury can be accomplished several years after the initial injury.

The authors have nothing to disclose.
[a] Division of Pediatric Rehabilitation Medicine, Department of Pediatrics, Rady Children's Hospital San Diego, University of California San Diego, 3020 Children's Way, MC 5096, San Diego, CA 92123, USA; [b] Division of Pediatric Respiratory Medicine, Department of Pediatrics, Rady Children's Hospital San Diego, University of California San Diego, 3020 Children's Way, San Diego, CA, USA; [c] Department of Physical Medicine and Rehabilitation, University of California Davis School of Medicine, 4860 Y Street, Sacramento, CA 95817, USA
* Corresponding author.
E-mail address: askalsky@rchsd.org

Phys Med Rehabil Clin N Am 26 (2015) 133–143
http://dx.doi.org/10.1016/j.pmr.2014.09.010
1047-9651/15/$ – see front matter © 2015 Elsevier Inc. All rights reserved.

INTRODUCTION: NATURE OF THE PROBLEM

A phrenic nerve pacing system consists of implanted receivers and electrodes, external antennas worn directly over the implanted receivers, and an external transmitter. The external transmitter and antennas send energy to the implanted receivers. The electrical stimulation is accomplished by transcutaneous radiofrequency stimulation of the implanted receivers by the external antennas. The implanted receivers receive the radiofrequency energy and convert it to electrical impulses, which directly stimulate the phrenic nerves. The phrenic nerve stimulation leads to contraction of the diaphragms (**Fig. 1**).

Electric stimulation of the phrenic nerve was first applied by Sarnoff and colleagues[1] in 1948 in the setting of ventilatory insufficiency. Glenn and colleagues[2] electrically stimulated the phrenic nerve through radiofrequency induction and successfully applied the technique clinically. Onders and colleagues[3,4] described a method of directly stimulating the diaphragm to achieve successful ventilation. Diaphragm pacing via phrenic nerve stimulation requires an intact phrenic nerve and a functioning diaphragm. Patients with primary neuropathies and myopathies are generally not good candidates for this therapy. In pediatric centers, diaphragm pacing has been most commonly used for patients with high cervical spinal cord injury and for those with central hypoventilation syndromes such as congenital central hypoventilation syndrome. Successful application of these techniques for patients with spinal cord injury requires careful evaluation of phrenic nerve and diaphragmatic function.

Fluoroscopy is used in many institutions to evaluate diaphragmatic motion in the setting of presumed diaphragmatic paralysis. Fluoroscopy is limited by the use of

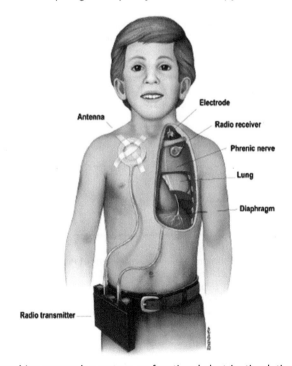

Fig. 1. Avery breathing pacemaker system, an functional electric stimulation system for respiratory muscles by phrenic nerve stimulation. (*Courtesy of* Avery Biomedical Devices, Inc., Commack, NY; with permission.)

ionizing radiation and the requirement for patient transport to a specialized examination or surgical suite. In addition, fluoroscopy provides qualitative images but cannot provide quantitative data regarding diaphragmatic motion.

Electrodiagnostic motor nerve conduction studies (mNCS) and electromyography (EMG) are conventionally used to evaluate the function and integrity of the phrenic nerve in the setting of diaphragmatic paralysis, but these methods possess several disadvantages. Phrenic nerve mNCS can be technically difficult to perform because of patients' body habitus and confounding electrical interference.[5,6] These factors can be especially limiting for a ventilated patient in an intensive care unit. In addition, mNCS only provide data regarding the phrenic nerve and corresponding diaphragmatic muscle action potentials, which serve as surrogate markers of phrenic nerve and diaphragmatic function. Phrenic nerve mNCS can be useful for detecting and quantifying the injury to the phrenic nerve, but the reliability and reproducibility are suboptimal.[5,6] Although mNCS have been used to determine eligibility for phrenic nerve and diaphragm pacing systems, they offer no direct measurement of diaphragmatic response to phrenic nerve stimulation.[7]

Performing EMG on the diaphragm can be daunting for an inexperienced electromyographer, owing to the small risk for pneumothorax.[8,9] Similarly to fluoroscopy, EMG of the diaphragm provides only qualitative data regarding spontaneous activity and motor unit recruitment. In the setting of partial axonotmesis, EMG is not able to assess for the presence of adequate axonal function to achieve sufficient stimulation of the diaphragm and attain adequate ventilation with phrenic nerve stimulation.

This report details one center's protocol for the assessment of diaphragmatic response to phrenic nerve stimulation. The technique provides information regarding the integrity of the phrenic nerve, anatomic etiology of diaphragmatic paralysis, and the potential for phrenic nerve pacing through transcutaneous stimulation of the phrenic nerve and direct visualization of the resulting diaphragmatic movement with ultrasonography. In addition to the initial evaluation for candidacy for phrenic nerve or diaphragmatic pacing systems, the utility of the technique for long-term follow-up and settings adjustments of the pacing systems are reviewed.

DESCRIPTION OF TECHNIQUE
Diaphragmatic Ultrasonography

Diaphragmatic ultrasonography is performed with the patient in the supine position. For the older pediatric and adult patient, a multifrequency 4-MHz vector transducer is used in the longitudinal semicoronal plane using a subcostal or low intercostal approach extending from the midaxillary to the midclavicular lines. In young pediatric patients, a multifrequency 7-MHz vector transducer is used from the same approach. The right diaphragm is visualized through the window of the liver, and the left diaphragm is visualized though the window of the spleen.[10]

Diaphragmatic ultrasonography provides direct visualization of the diaphragm, qualitative evaluation of diaphragmatic excursion, and quantitative evaluation of diaphragmatic motion with M-mode ultrasonography. M-mode sonography allows for quantification of diaphragmatic motion by recording the successive positions of the diaphragm in relation to time. Patients are initially examined with and without mechanically assisted ventilation (**Figs. 2** and **3**). The ventilator is temporarily disconnected when the patient undergoes phrenic nerve stimulation.

Phrenic Nerve Stimulation

Several techniques have been described for phrenic nerve stimulation.[5–7] The authors routinely stimulate at the posterior border of the sternocleidomastoid (SCM) sternal

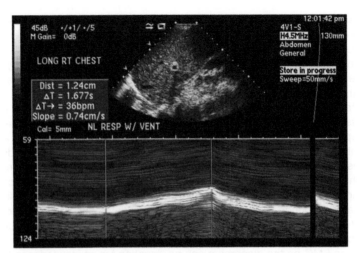

Fig. 2. M-mode diaphragm ultrasonography while on mechanical ventilation.

head and anterior to the clavicular heads of the SCM muscle just above the clavicle. The SCM muscles can be made more prominent by having the patient flex the neck for a few seconds to aid in positioning of the stimulator. A bipolar surface electrode stimulator is used for the phrenic nerve stimulations. The current required for supramaximal stimulation is usually less than 50 mA. The stimulation can be provided by the bipolar stimulator of a traditional electrodiagnostic device.

Evaluation of Phrenic Nerve Function

Patients with diaphragmatic paralysis can be evaluated for a positive or negative response to phrenic nerve stimulation. A positive response is characterized by the detection of a spike-like deflection with M-mode ultrasonography after phrenic nerve stimulation (**Fig. 4**). This diaphragmatic motion in response to phrenic nerve

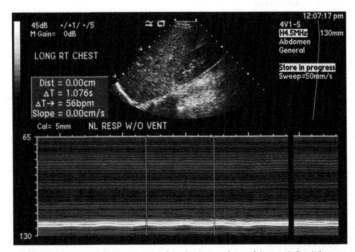

Fig. 3. M-mode diaphragm ultrasonography during a breathing trial without mechanical ventilation in an individual with no spontaneous respirations. Note the flat line indicating no movement.

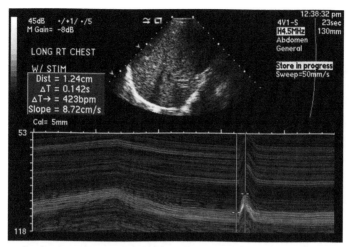

Fig. 4. M-mode diaphragm ultrasonography after transcutaneous phrenic nerve stimulation, with a spike deflection indicating a positive response.

stimulation represents partial or complete continuity of the phrenic nerve and candidacy for phrenic nerve pacing. In the setting of complete axonotmesis of the phrenic nerve, no diaphragmatic motion is detected. Both the left and right phrenic nerves and corresponding hemidiaphragms can and should be studied independently. It should be noted that evaluation of the phrenic nerves should be delayed for a minimum of 72 hours in the setting of trauma to prevent a false-positive result arising from incomplete wallerian degeneration of the phrenic nerve axons.

M-mode ultrasonography can also be implemented in the initial titration of a phrenic nerve or diaphragmatic pacing system. The alternative method of ventilation should be discontinued before initiation of phrenic nerve pacing. Each phrenic nerve and corresponding hemidiaphragm is initially evaluated independent of the contralateral side. The amplitude control on the external transmitter is slowly increased until the maximum diaphragmatic excursion measured by M-mode ultrasonography is reached (**Fig. 5**). This process should be repeated for the contralateral phrenic nerve and corresponding hemidiaphragm with the initial side unpaced. Concomitant measurements of hemidiaphragm tidal volumes can be measured using a spirometer. If the patient has a tracheostomy, the cuff needs to be inflated to ensure minimal air leak, which would artificially decrease the measured hemidiaphragm tidal volume. Once the optimal stimulation amplitude has been established, the rate can be adjusted based on sequential clinical evaluations, pulse oximetry, capnography, tidal volume measurement, calculated minute ventilation, and ultimately arterial blood gas (ABG) measurements. Reassessment of the pacing stimulation amplitude with M-mode diaphragmatic ultrasonography and/or spirometry should be performed yearly, as should reassessment of the stimulation rate.

CASE REPORTS
Case 1

J.O. sustained a C1 ASIA A spinal cord transection in a pedestrian versus automobile accident at 7 years of age with resulting complete diaphragm paralysis. He was initially ventilated with positive pressure via tracheostomy in the critical care setting. J.O. underwent bilateral phrenic nerve evaluations with transcutaneous nerve stimulation

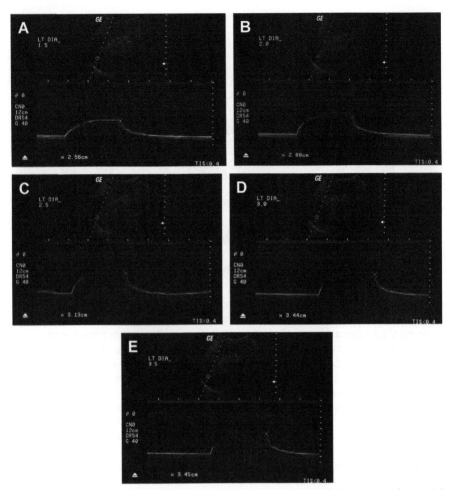

Fig. 5. (A) M-mode diaphragm ultrasonography with pacer amplitude setting of 1.5, with resulting diaphragm excursion of 2.56 cm. (B) M-mode diaphragm ultrasonography with pacer amplitude setting of 2.0, with resulting diaphragm excursion of 2.88 cm. (C) M-mode diaphragm ultrasonography with pacer amplitude setting of 2.5, with resulting diaphragm excursion of 3.13 cm. (D) M-mode diaphragm ultrasonography with pacer amplitude setting of 3.0, with resulting diaphragm excursion of 3.44 cm. (E) M-mode diaphragm ultrasonography with pacer amplitude setting of 3.5, with resulting diaphragm excursion of 3.45 cm.

and diaphragmatic ultrasonography as described. A positive response was obtained and, 35 days following the injury, bilateral phrenic nerve pacers were implanted in the cervical region. Two weeks after implantation of the system, pacing was initiated at 30-minute intervals and was gradually titrated. Within 2 months, J.O. was able to use 24-hour pacing. J.O. continued to use 4 hours per day of bilevel positive airway pressure (BPAP) via tracheostomy nocturnally. Based on observation, the inspiratory cycle of the bilevel device was triggered by the phrenic nerve pacing device. The treating team's main goal of positive airway pressure therapy for this patient centered on avoidance of atelectasis. After pacer placement, J.O. had one hospitalization for pneumonia over a 13-year time span. He underwent baclofen pump placement for spasticity management, posterior spinal fusion for neurogenic scoliosis, and cystolithotomy for bladder calculi. J.O. has graduated from high school as the class valedictorian.

Case 2

H.L. sustained a C2 ASIA A spinal cord injury from a gunshot wound to the right neck at 15 years of age. A tracheostomy was placed near the time of the accident, and he was ventilated via a positive pressure ventilator. H.L. then underwent bilateral phrenic nerve evaluation with transcutaneous nerve stimulation and diaphragmatic ultrasonography as described. A positive response was obtained on the left and a negative response on the right. It was therefore assumed that the right phrenic nerve or its nuclei within the anterior horn cells of the spinal cord were significantly damaged during the initial trauma. Approximately 6 months following injury, the phrenic nerve pacing system was implanted bilaterally into the neck by an otolaryngologist (**Fig. 6**). Two weeks after implantation of the system, bilateral pacing was initiated. With both pacer sides active, the left hemidiaphragm demonstrated normal excursion (**Fig. 7**A), and there was paradoxic movement of the right hemidiaphragm. With only the right-side pacer activated, trace right diaphragmatic excursion was observed on ultrasonography (see **Fig. 7**B). Four months later, H.L. was using diaphragm pacing for 24 hours per day while using BPAP via tracheostomy for 6 hours during sleep with the goal of minimizing atelectasis. Since pacer placement, H.L. has had only one pulmonary-related hospitalization for right whole lung atelectasis secondary to mucus plugging in the setting of an upper respiratory infection. She has also undergone baclofen pump placement for spasticity management. H.L. has been successfully treated primarily using the phrenic nerve pacing system augmented by positive pressure ventilation via tracheostomy during a portion of sleep for more than 9 years, despite unilateral phrenic nerve injury with resulting diaphragm paralysis not amenable to functional pacing.

Case 3

L.B. sustained a C3 ASIA A spinal cord injury from a diving accident at 11 years of age. L.B. was dependent on a mechanical ventilator via tracheostomy for the first 2 years following the injury. L.B. then underwent bilateral diaphragmatic ultrasonography and

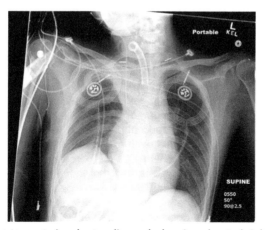

Fig. 6. Standard posteroanterior chest radiograph showing elevated right hemidiaphragm and phrenic nerve pacing antenna leads.

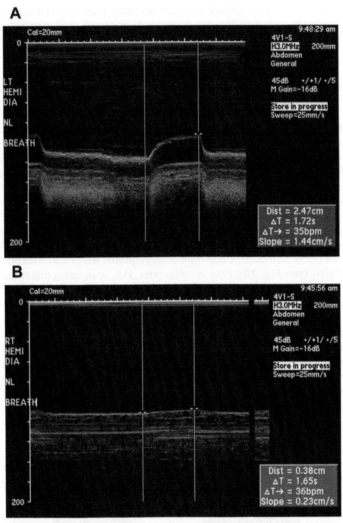

Fig. 7. (A) Left diaphragmatic motion of patient H.L. with phrenic nerve pacing system. (B) Right diaphragmatic motion of patient H.L. with phrenic nerve pacing system.

phrenic nerve evaluations with transcutaneous nerve stimulation as described. The left hemidiaphragm demonstrated normal spontaneous excursion with spontaneous breathing; however, there was slight paradoxic increase of the right hemidiaphragm during inspiration. With transcutaneous right phrenic nerve stimulation a positive response to simulation was observed, with the usual spike deflection with M-mode ultrasonography. It was concluded that L.B.'s left phrenic nerve and hemidiaphragm had adequate spontaneous function, but that the right was paralyzed. L.B. elected to undergo implantation of a right-sided phrenic nerve pacing system. Within 1 month of initiating pacing, L.B. was using the diaphragmatic pacing system for 24 hours per day while continuing nocturnal positive pressure ventilation via BPAP during part of sleep. Before placement of the right phrenic nerve pacer, L.B. was hospitalized on 4 occasions for respiratory infection. After placement of the phrenic nerve pacing system, L.B. had 13 years without a hospitalization for respiratory-related infection. L.B. has also tolerated 3 baclofen pump placements without postoperative respiratory complication since transitioning to unilateral phrenic nerve pacing.

Case 4

At 7 years of age Z.B. sustained a C2 ASIA A spinal cord injury resulting from an accident involving a dirt bike and an automobile, with resulting diaphragm paralysis and mechanical ventilator dependence. More than 4 years after his injury, Z.B. was evaluated for eligibility of a phrenic nerve pacing system using the technique described. After only 2 months of a graduated schedule of phrenic nerve pacing accompanied by intermittent mechanical ventilation, Z.B. successfully achieved day-time ventilation with only the phrenic nerve pacing system, despite being more than 4 years removed from the initial injury.

DISCUSSION

Diaphragmatic paralysis can lead to inadequate breathing and chronic respiratory failure with requirement for ventilatory support. Assisted ventilation may be achieved by using positive pressure devices via tracheostomy or mask interfaces, negative pressure devices such as the iron lung or cuirass, or phrenic nerve and diaphragm pacing. Phrenic nerve or diaphragm pacing exists as a desirable modality for the treatment of chronic respiratory failure in the appropriate setting, owing to the ability of affected individuals to breathe independently of mechanical ventilation.

Phrenic motor nerve conduction studies and diaphragmatic electromyography have been used to determine the integrity of the phrenic nerve in the setting of diaphragmatic paralysis. In comparison with traditional phrenic mNCS, which record the compound muscle action potential (CMAP) of the diaphragm using surface electrodes, ultrasonographic evaluation of the diaphragm with phrenic nerve stimulation provides direct observation of diaphragmatic movement in response to phrenic nerve stimulation. In addition, mNCS results can be technically influenced by concomitant brachial plexus stimulation, which can lead to a false-positive finding. Such a false-positive finding could result in the implantation of phrenic nerve or diaphragm pacing system that will ultimately fail. With direct observation of diaphragmatic movement with ultrasonography, concomitant brachial plexus stimulation will not alter the findings. However, CMAP onset latency in traditional phrenic nerve conduction studies are more useful in detecting demyelination of the phrenic nerves if a demyelinating process is suspected, but mNCS still do not offer the same amount of clinical information regarding the potential for phrenic nerve or diaphragm pacing candidacy.

Phrenic nerve pacing has many advantages over positive pressure ventilation, including a more physiologic negative pressure ventilation. Hirschfeld and colleagues[11] reported a lower incidence of respiratory infections and improved quality of speech. A significant percentage of affected individuals reports preference of phrenic nerve pacing over mechanical ventilation.

Several modalities have been used to determine if and to what extent the diaphragm is paralyzed. Plain-film radiography and fluoroscopy are most commonly used. Fluoroscopy has traditionally been used and continues to be so in many institutions to assess diaphragmatic motion. There are several disadvantages to using fluoroscopy, including ionizing radiation and the requirement to transport the patient to the fluoroscopy equipment. Conversely, ultrasonography requires no radiation and can be performed at the patient's bedside. A comparison study of ultrasonography and fluoroscopy in the assessment of diaphragmatic motion found no technical failure with ultrasonography, and an 81% agreement between both modalities. Ultrasonography revealed all abnormalities that were seen on fluoroscopy. Conversely, ultrasonography was more sensitive to motion than fluoroscopy.[12] Ultrasonographic evaluation of diaphragm motion is an accurate, reliable technique that is widely available. The primary limitations of ultrasonography are the inability to simultaneously image both hemidiaphragms and the technique being operator dependent. The authors therefore suggest ultrasonography as the modality of choice in the examination of motion of the diaphragm because it is portable, readily available, and uses no ionizing radiation.[10]

Management of individuals using diaphragmatic pacing systems requires ongoing care with access to a center with expertise in the management of patients with chronic respiratory failure. Although strategies to care for patients with diaphragm pacing vary across practitioners, most aim to normalize oxygenation and ventilation, minimize atelectasis and pneumonia, and increase the quality of life. After initial placement of diaphragmatic pacers, some experts wait 1 to 4 weeks before initiating pacing to allow for surgical wound healing and minimize the frequent setting changes that may occur as scar tissue forms around the transmitter.[13] Pacing is sometimes first initiated for 60 to 90 minutes per day and is slowly increased over weeks to months. It has been the authors' practice to use diaphragm pacers in pediatric patients without the addition of positive pressure ventilation for a maximum of 12 to 20 hours per day. Positive pressure ventilation is often added overnight via tracheostomy and ventilator to reduce atelectasis. The benefit of concomitant use of positive pressure ventilation with diaphragm pacing has not been well described.

Once pacing is initiated, an amplitude and rate are chosen to approximate the patient's minute ventilation. The respiratory rate is generally chosen based on the patient's age and corresponding physiologic frequency of breathing. It is recommended that pacing generally be initiated either in the inpatient setting or in a sleep laboratory with expertise in diaphragm pacing, especially for pediatric patients with abnormal ventilatory control or effort. Ultrasonography can be used to subjectively assess diaphragmatic excursion during pacing initiation. If ultrasonography is not readily available, contraction of the diaphragms and chest rise can often be observed through palpation of the abdominal wall, and visualization of symmetric chest and abdominal movement during pacing. Measuring carbon dioxide levels with end-tidal, transcutaneous, and/or blood gas techniques can be used to monitor ventilation. A pneumotach may be helpful in patients who have cuffed tracheostomies to measure tidal volume and flow. Although goal carbon dioxide values vary across centers, many aim for normal to low levels. The benefits of mild hyperventilation with CO_2 levels of 30 to 40 mm Hg include hypothetical allowance for a reserve in patients managed in the home.[13] This approach can be especially pertinent in the setting of respiratory infection, diminished airway clearance, and variability with changes in sleep position and sleep stage.

In addition, it is recommended that oxygenation be measured and monitored, accomplished most often through pulse oximetry. Goal oxygen saturations are generally greater than 93% to 95%. Continuous oximetry can be not only applied as a test of adequacy of diaphragm pacer settings but also used as an alarm in the setting of device malfunction. However, hypoventilation can occur in the setting of normal or near normal oxygen saturation. Thus, pulse oximetry should not be considered a substitute for intermittent monitoring of ventilation through measurement of carbon dioxide levels.

After pacing is established, patients should have diaphragm pacer and positive pressure device settings monitored periodically. Ideally this occurs via overnight polysomnography or during an inpatient admission for titration. The potential benefits of polysomnography include continuous monitoring of gas exchange, identification of obstructive and central sleep apnea, and ensuring adequate breathing across all sleep stages and positions. Regardless of the overall ventilatory strategy used to initiate and maintain adequate respiration with diaphragm pacing, practitioners should anticipate the need for frequent attention and be prepared to be flexible, collaborative, and creative as problems arise.

REFERENCES

1. Sarnoff SJ, Hardenbergh E, Whittenberger JL. Electrophrenic respiration. Am J Physiol 1948;155(1):1–9.
2. Glenn WW, Holcomb WG, McLaughlin AJ, et al. Total ventilatory support in a quadriplegic patient with radiofrequency electrophrenic respiration. N Engl J Med 1972;286(10):513–6.
3. DiMarco AF, Onders RP, Kowalski KE, et al. Phrenic nerve pacing in a tetraplegic patient via intramuscular diaphragm electrodes. Am J Respir Crit Care Med 2002; 166(12 Pt 1):1604–6.
4. Onders RP, DiMarco AF, Ignagni AR, et al. Mapping the phrenic nerve motor point: the key to a successful laparoscopic diaphragm pacing system in the first human series. Surgery 2004;136(4):819–26.
5. Resman-Gaspersc A, Podnar S. Phrenic nerve conduction studies: technical aspects and normative data. Muscle Nerve 2008;37(1):36–41.
6. Chen R, Collins S, Remtulla H, et al. Phrenic nerve conduction study in normal subjects. Muscle Nerve 1995;18(3):330–5.
7. Alshekhlee A, Onders RP, Syed TU, et al. Phrenic nerve conduction studies in spinal cord injury: applications for diaphragmatic pacing. Muscle Nerve 2008; 38(6):1546–52.
8. Bolton CF. AAEM minimonograph #40: clinical neurophysiology of the respiratory system [review]. Muscle Nerve 1993;16(8):809–18.
9. Podnar S. Pneumothorax after needle electromyography of the diaphragm: a case report. Neurol Sci 2013;34:1243–5.
10. Gerscovich EO, Cronan M, McGahan JP, et al. Ultrasonographic evaluation of diaphragmatic motion. J Ultrasound Med 2001;20(6):597–604.
11. Hirschfeld S, Exner G, Luukkaala T, et al. Mechanical ventilation or phrenic nerve stimulation for treatment of spinal cord injury-induced respiratory insufficiency. Spinal Cord 2008;46(11):738–42. http://dx.doi.org/10.1038/sc.2008.43.
12. Houston JG, Fleet M, Cowan MD, et al. Comparison of ultrasound with fluoroscopy in the assessment of suspected hemidiaphragmatic movement abnormality. Clin Radiol 1995;50(2):95–8.
13. Chen MD, Tablizo MA, Kun S, et al. Diaphragm pacers as a treatment for congenital central hypoventilation syndrome. Expert Rev Med Devices 2005;2(5):577–85.

Index

Note: Page numbers of article titles are in **boldface** type.

A

Above-knee amputations, 104
Accelerometer, ankle-worn, for K-level determination, 105
Accident prevention education, 101
Accidents. See *Traumatic entries.*
Actin, in muscle force production, 58–59
Action potential, compound muscle, of diaphragm, 141
Acupuncture, for hypertonicity, 71
Adam forward-bend test, for scoliosis, 22
Adolescents, disabled, caregiving for, 9–12
	factors of living, 13–14
Adult care, disabled adolescents transitioning to, 9–12
	functional factors of, 13–14
	for spina bifida patients, **29–38**
		epidemiology of, 29–30
		interest in, 30–31
		introduction to, 29
		key points of, 29
		multisystem conditions in, 31–35
			cognitive care, 34
			gastrointestinal care, 34
			living concerns, 35
			neurosurgical care, 32
			orthopedic care, 33
			physiatry care, 34
			physical medicine, 34
			primary care, 31–32
			psychological care, 34–35
			rehabilitation, 34
			social concerns, 35
			urologic care, 32–33
			vocational concerns, 35
			women's health, 35
		summary overview of, 36
		transitional care in, 31
		transitional program for, 35–36
Adulthood, disabled adolescents transition to, 9–12
	functional factors of, 13–14
Age/aging, growth percentile per, for cerebral palsy children, 48
	of disabled adolescents, 9–12
	pediatric neuromuscular disorders and, 25
Alcohol abuse, in caregivers, 8

Phys Med Rehabil Clin N Am 26 (2015) 145–173
http://dx.doi.org/10.1016/S1047-9651(14)00131-4
1047-9651/15/$ – see front matter © 2015 Elsevier Inc. All rights reserved.

pmr.theclinics.com

Moving?

Make sure your subscription moves with you!

To notify us of your new address, find your **Clinics Account Number** (located on your mailing label above your name), and contact customer service at:

Email: journalscustomerservice-usa@elsevier.com

800-654-2452 (subscribers in the U.S. & Canada)
314-447-8871 (subscribers outside of the U.S. & Canada)

Fax number: 314-447-8029

Elsevier Health Sciences Division
Subscription Customer Service
3251 Riverport Lane
Maryland Heights, MO 63043

*To ensure uninterrupted delivery of your subscription,
please notify us at least 4 weeks in advance of move.

Printed and bound by CPI Group (UK) Ltd, Croydon, CR0 4YY

03/10/2024

01040490-0018